How Walking Saved My Life

Heather Waring

Dedication

To Alan and Ellie who had no choice but to come on this journey with me and who continue to have my back.

Acknowledgements

I have been so lucky to have many great people on this journey with me, including the women I have had the pleasure to walk with through these years and those I now have the pleasure to lead on Camino Experiences and other walk adventures.

I'd like to specifically thank Frea O'Brien who gave me a very firm deadline to work to; Ale Buljevich for her beautiful cover shot and back cover head shot; Julie Stevens for the book cover design; Fiona Lafferty my editor, who inspired me as she edited and my mentors along this way Joanna Martin, Fabienne Fredrickson and Julie Creffield.

Finally to my amazing Evolve Mastermind of Gail Morgan, Julie Stevens and Karen Knott. Love you all.

Foreward

How could something as simple as putting one foot in front of the other be a life-saver? This incredible book will explain exactly why walking is so powerful and will give you both inspiration and enjoyment.

No-one has to convince me of the benefits of exercise, but there is far more to walking than simply getting fit. Heather's story about how walking came to her physical and emotional rescue is one that many, many people will resonate with and appreciate. The story is not just about how walking had a massive impact on her life - it is about how it can have a massive impact on the life of almost anyone - and you already have everything you need for it to benefit you too.

Heather has this wonderful skill of supporting women to be the best versions of themselves. Through her own life experiences, storytelling skills and ability to make sense of the world, she helps others do the same in their own lives.

I feel honoured to have been part of the conception of Heather's *One Million Women Walking* campaign, which despite its already phenomenal growth I know is only at the start of its development, and I am humbled to have been asked to write this foreword.

This book is a significant marker for Heather as she takes an even bigger step into her global leadership role. I am sure that reading it will be a significant step for you too.

Enjoy the journey!

Julie Creffield, London, January 2020

Solvitur ambulando -
It is solved by walking.

(often attributed to St Augustine)

THE PAST

Chapter 1

'Please don't develop any further, please don't develop into a cold'.

I repeated silently to myself. I was addressing the dry, tickly feeling at the back of my throat that had been present for days. These words became like a mantra in my head as I worked on; knowing, as I was saying them, that if I were to stop and give myself a break all would be better. But there was work to finish and it had to be done before I went on holiday.

I was working across time zones, organising interviews, finalising dates for blog publications and generally negotiating publicity for a virtual book tour. Each day started at 8.00 a.m. and went on till around midnight, and I'd been doing this for too many days now without a break. I knew I was pushing myself too hard, but I had a 9-day holiday coming up so I figured that if I could just get to that point, I could rest. To have all these interviews and dates for article and blog publication set up before I went away, meant flow and ease when I returned.

Since this time, that dry tickly feeling has become my warning sign. Whenever I feel it, I know I am pushing a little too far and I step back.

Perhaps, if I'd been going to lay by a pool in the sun, I could have stopped the tsunami that was headed my way, but at this moment I had no idea what might befall me.

I was heading off to France to walk another section of the Camino de Santiago, continuing the journey I had started in 2008 in Le Puy en Velay in the Massive Central area. This was my 1000-mile journey on the iconic pilgrimage path walked by so many over hundreds of years, and now undergoing a great resurgence, attracting modern-day pilgrims from all over the world.

Unable to do what the majority do, which is to start in St Jean and walk 500 miles (800 km) to Santiago over 4–6 weeks, my walking buddy and I had decided to start in the centre of France, thereby doubling the length of our walk. We would cover the miles by walking a section (around 75 -90 miles) that would take about a week each year.

We were about to start our second half, and the most popular bit. We were approaching the French/Spanish border and this section, starting in the pretty little town of St Jean Pied de Port in the Pyrenean foothills, would take us up and over the Pyrenees. From there we would walk on to Logroño, the capital of the province of La Rioja in Northern Spain, a distance of around 100 miles/162 km.

This section over the Pyrenees is one of the most challenging, and we had carefully chosen mid-September. Our thinking was that the snow would not yet have arrived, the paths would be clear and dry after the summer months, and we would hopefully have great views. Sadly, we arrived in St Jean in rain, and it was still raining the next morning as, backpacks and waterproofs on, we joined many others at the Pilgrim Office to collect our passport for our journey.

Your Pilgrim passport (Credencial del Peregrino) is a record of your journey. You collect 'stamps' at the places you stay, in some of the churches, and in many of the bars and restaurants. If you want to claim your Pilgrim Certificate, your Compostella, once you get to Santiago, you must walk at least the last 100 kms of this path into Santiago and have at least two stamps a day. If you start from outside Galicia, then you must have at least one a day – but in my experience, you will want to collect many more. These stamps are so individual to the places you get them, and once you're back home, they bring back such wonderful memories of the people who stamped your passport and the places you gathered them. In France, the passport is not often used, and passport stamps are few and far between, so for us being able to have our passport was very significant. It can also often get you reduced rates in museums and other places of interest along the way.

There was a real buzz of activity in the Pilgrim Office and I could immediately feel myself getting caught up in the excitement. There were so many people chatting and laughing, so many different languages, and so many conversations regarding destinations, timescales and plans. Even though we had already been walking this path for many years, this was a whole new experience for us and we were excited to see it unfold.

It was still raining as we left the building but, with passports safely tucked where the damp would not reach and water bottles full, we were raring to get going. The path continued down the steep cobbled street, across the Pilgrim bridge and then, of course, up. We had no real idea what was ahead of us, we just knew that the time had come to go over the mountains, those we had seen ahead of us on many previous sections.

The weather didn't improve as the day went on. Up and up we trudged along a road that just seemed to get steeper and steeper. For some reason, I had assumed that after a while we would have been walking on grassy tracks or on earthen paths that would have been so much easier on our feet, but it was not to be. I was grateful for my comfortable shoes, well tested over many miles, and I was also grateful I wasn't on a bike! For the many cyclists, the downs might be fun, but on this part of the journey they seemed to be peddling away and making little progress. However, everyone was jovial, and there was always someone to speak to and to laugh with, and to share comments about the challenge of the path as we questioned why on earth we were doing this.

I always feel it's important to stop and look to see from whence you have come. If you don't, you run the risk of missing out on the great vistas behind you. It's also a good excuse for a short rest and a chance to catch your breath, but on this particular day there were no views to be had. The mist had rolled in, and the higher we went, the denser it became and the colder it was too. The road went on and on.

The refuge Orisson came into view after only 5 miles/8 kms, but as it was hours since we had set off, it felt we had done at least twice that distance! What a welcome sight. This is the only stopping place on the way to Roncesvalles and, with a mere 18 beds, gets booked up well in advance. We were not looking for a bed, just a coffee (and on this occasion a piece of Tarte de Santiago) and a stamp for our passport. It was a blissful 30 minutes of rest, drinking in the atmosphere, watching people come and go and again hearing so many different languages spoken. When we could eke out this time in this warm and cosy place no longer, it was time to pull on wet outer clothes again, hoist the backpack onto our shoulders and get back on the path.

One of the marker points on this section is a statue of the Virgin at Biakorre.

From here, the views on a good day stretch for miles, but so dense was the mist that we missed this completely. The Virgin? What virgin? I had to wait until 2018, when I walked this section again with an American friend, to see the Virgin and experience the absolute beauty and stunning scenery of this part of the path. On that occasion we sat in the sunshine having lunch and watching the eagles and other birds of prey soaring above and below us. It was worth every step of the ups to see just what I had missed before.

Finally, off the road about an hour later we had to search carefully for markers and the ground under our feet was uneven and very muddy in places – so much for the experience we had envisaged. We even missed the sign that we had crossed the border into Spain, so the small bottles of Cava we had carried to celebrate this important event stayed in our rucksacks.

The path became much flatter, and there was a fountain so we could refill our bottles. Life felt like it was looking up – forgive the pun. Perhaps we had finished with the ups! No such luck. Back on the road again further along and more climbing, all be it not as steep, but still it seemed relentless and, as we looked ahead, there was no sign of it stopping. At last, we reached a signpost with many different directions suggested, and other signs telling us that in bad weather the most direct path down into Roncesvalles was not advised. Much as we wanted to take it, sense did prevail, as the last thing we needed was for one of us to fall and sustain a serious injury. It felt like many hours later when we trudged into the small village that was to be our home for the night.

There is much history caught up in this small place, and today much of that is to do with the monastery and the fact that this is a major place on the Camino. We had booked accommodation in advance, something for which we were extremely grateful, as we were aware of the number of walkers we had chatted to on our journey and who were still behind us who were hoping to find a bed once they arrived. We were informed when we checked in that all beds had been filled by 4.30 and it was now about 7.00. I did wonder where they would all sleep.

The bar in our small hotel was very busy and there were no seats, but upstairs we discovered a lounge area and here, better late than never, we toasted the crossing into Spain and the completion of a very long, wet day, as we lay cosy and warm, on soft, roomy sofas…the worst, we felt, was over.

As we set off on Day 2, the rain was a constant companion. We walked on a path through the trees, the ground under our feet sodden, and the drips from the trees bouncing off our hoods. Then, suddenly in the afternoon it stopped, the clouds cleared, and the sun came out.

Over the next few days it became very hot. The pendulum had swung wildly, so from wearing gloves as we crossed the mountains, we were now walking in temperatures of 35 degrees! On many of the paths shade was hard to find, and even though we drank plenty of water, wore high-factor sunscreen and brimmed hats, walked in shade where possible and rested regularly, it was tough going. By 2.00 in the afternoon it really felt like we were walking in a furnace! It was so hot at night that neither of us slept, and it was a welcome break to sometimes start our days before sunrise just so we could minimise the afternoon walking.

What a relief to reach Logroño on our final day, collapse into a chair at a café in the square and order the celebratory large beers that brought to an end one of the most challenging walks I'd undertaken. Even with the heat, it had been beautiful. I loved Pamplona with its beautiful cathedral, the ancient streets of the old town and the walls of the city. Walking up to the Alto de Perdon, roughly translated as Hill of Forgiveness was a defining moment. On this hill is a beautiful steel sculpture of pilgrims on their route to Santiago. Erected in 1996, it's one of the most iconic symbols of the Camino and I had seen its image so often. I also loved the pilgrim bridge at Puente La Reina.

I do remember feeling exhausted at the airport, more so than usual, but then it had been a challenging trip. When we arrived at the bus station back in Stansted there were long queues and a lack of buses. There had been an accident on the motorway, so those buses not caught up in that were having to take an alternative, cross-country route. Tempers were frayed and I was really fed up; I just wanted to get home. When the bus did arrive, the journey was long, twisty and of the kind that makes your stomach churn. I was feeling really irritable and was trying hard not to snap. I put it all down to tiredness.

That evening my darling husband, Alan, looked after me, providing dinner, tending to my every need, and being patient with my wish to say little. I was early to bed, sleeping well; was it only the bliss of own bed or my total exhaustion? Probably both and it didn't matter.

"It's your road, and yours alone.
Others may walk it with you,
but no one can walk it for you."
– Rumi

Chapter 2

The next morning seemed normal enough. Alan had let me sleep, so, bleary eyed, I padded downstairs and into the kitchen to find breakfast. What did I want? I hadn't a clue.... What I couldn't be bothered doing was making my usual green juice; it was too much hassle. I wanted something quick, so resorted to Shreddies and banana and took myself into the lounge. Three hours later, I was still there watching mindless TV.

Now this is not me, but I was still feeling so tired. I put it all down to that and allowed myself to go back to bed. I slept, but felt no better on waking and never quite managed to get dressed that day at all. If Alan was concerned, he didn't show it. I still wasn't talking much; I couldn't be bothered. Everything seemed too hard. Tomorrow would be better... but it wasn't.

The third day dawned, and with it the continued malaise of being fed up, not caring what happened with anything. Decisions were hard to make, so, as much as possible, I didn't make them. I just ate what was put in front of me. I was still sleeping loads and I was still not getting dressed or at least not until late afternoon. I was also very tearful, and I didn't have a clue why. Tears flowed at all sorts of moments, gushing, sobbing and at some points even howling, but I kept that to myself as much as possible.

At this point, Alan was concerned, and so was I. Yes, I'd done a long walk under difficult conditions, but I'd still enjoyed it. However, I'd done walks of this length and difficulty before and all had been well. Yes, I'd had little sleep while away, but I couldn't kick this feeling of doom like a black cloud hanging over me. I am generally a pretty high-energy, upbeat person, and this was as far away from that as I had ever been. There was nothing I wanted to do and nowhere I wanted to be.

Insight came from an unexpected source. I picked up my battered copy of 'Simple Abundance' that afternoon – it was 1st October – and I read the segment for that day. It was entitled 'Recognising Burnout Before You're Charred', and there was a quote from Edna St Vincent Millay which said, "My candle burns at both ends; it will not last the night." Already I was feeling something.

I read on, every word awakening a realisation within.
Let me share a little with you -

"It's burnout when you go to bed exhausted every night and wake up tired every morning – when no amount of sleep refreshes you month after weary month. It's burnout when everything becomes too much effort: combing your hair, going out to dinner, visiting friends for the weekend, even going on

vacation. ...It's burnout when you find yourself cranky all the time, bursting into tears or going into fits of rage at the slightest provocation."

I read on, the mist in my mind clearing and reality starting to peak through. I had burnt out!

At least I knew what was wrong and that was a great relief. I grabbed my book and rushed down to the office thrusting it in front of Alan and signalling that he should read. "So, what are you going to do?" my husband asked. Take some time off, was my reply. Take the rest of the year off was his. I did.......sort of.

I spent the first week allowing myself to sleep and to watch films while lying on the sofa, but after that I began to get bored. This was a good sign, but with it came another realisation – I had been here before. I began to see a pattern – times in the past, perhaps not so acutely but it was familiar – and I knew that this was when I would normally jump back in again. Taking a day or two always helped, but then I had jumped back in and just gone on as I had before, because I believed it was all ok again.

Hindsight is a great thing and, looking at these situations now, I realised that my behaviour, where I had more or less put on a plaster and kept going, played a major part in where I was now. This time, if I wanted to change things, I really had to exercise caution and not repeat this pattern.

I felt a mixture of emotions, on one hand pleased that I knew what was happening, and yet on the other scared and nervous. How do I put this right? What do I do? Do I just need time out? I hadn't a clue.

The more I sat with all of this, the more things started to make sense. So many instances of behaviour and feelings rose to the surface. All the times I had been irritable and quick to anger; where there was no one able to do things but me, so I didn't delegate because I was always disappointed that things weren't done as I wanted; me not sleeping well – tossing and turning in bed, my head full of things…mainly all those things I hadn't done yet and/or needed to attend to soon. I was so unhappy but wasn't sure why.

For months, perhaps even years, if I was honest with myself, I had felt lost and disconnected. I had lain awake in the early hours sobbing silently, afraid to wake my husband because what could he do? Some of the times, my tears were of anger towards him but mostly frustration at my lack of being unable to fix this. All of this, though, was also peppered with times when things were good, and when that happened, I would think it was all ok again. But the periods of joy never lasted long enough.

The other constant, both in the dark of the night and in moments of despair during the day was "What right did I have to be unhappy and ungrateful? Didn't I have a wonderful husband, a gorgeous daughter, we were all healthy. I had a home, there was money coming in, my daughter was doing well at school, we travelled, had great friends etc. So, what right did I have to feel this way? So many people have such terrible lives, my life was nowhere like that."

I had lost my zest, my spark, and with that my essence. I was losing my identity. I was scared, I wanted it back, but I couldn't see how. I didn't know what to do. I didn't know who to talk to. I couldn't see a way of finding 'me' ever again and that brought such a huge wave of sadness over me. It made me shake with fear.

My eyes were opening to what had been happening, but I still didn't know who to turn to. I read what I could get my hands on and practically, as I had decided, I cleared my diary apart from a few ongoing commitments.

One of these was my Athena networking. Although I was unclear where I was going – in all honesty I'd been unsure for a while – I was chairing the group and helping the regional director with the network training and other bits and pieces, so I felt that I was able to give. Ironic really, as one of the reasons us women get into that overwhelmed, busy, stressed place is because of always giving to others and not giving to ourselves! By giving, though, I had a purpose, one that I could do easily. I had the support of my fellow Athena ladies and I belonged, and all of this was very important at this moment in time. I could also put on a very convincing mask and perform. The mask was there in many areas of life and had been for so long. When it was on, it served me well and many had no idea of the turmoil going on. But did it really serve me? Authenticity is so important to me, but I wasn't being authentic. I can see that now. I was denying 'me' and who I was. I wasn't asking for help. I wasn't even admitting an issue or a problem.

How many of us are doing exactly the same thing? Hiding behind a mask because we have to, at least we think we have to. Pushing on and 'being' that person because things need doing, people depend on us and they need us. Not asking for help because that's being weak isn't it? I mean, we should be able to do this ourselves, shouldn't we?

Alan would sometimes ask me what I would say to a client I was working with who was facing what I was? I was of course able to provide many suggestions, to talk about how I would support them, and to help them see that asking for help was not weak but actually a strength. I could not do this for me, though, it was far too close. If I am honest, I was also ashamed and embarrassed about getting myself into this place.

The other thing that was a constant was my Mastermind group. I had known these women for years and this was a safe place for me to be open and vulnerable and to receive love, care and support. As our meetings were every six weeks, they weren't too frequent, and I could use the group for clarity and exploration because I really needed to find me again and as importantly and crucially find what I wanted to do.

I now call these my 'wilderness years'. They'd been around for quite a while, and at the time I had no idea as to what was unfolding. The not being able to get clarity on what I wanted to do or who I wanted to be was a big clue, but I didn't see it.

These years had started when my initial attempt at bringing walking into my business hadn't worked as I'd hoped. After a couple of years working on and testing all elements, I had to look at it as a serious business model and accept that it wasn't going to bring in the income I wanted. Not wanting to return to career coaching, I had worked very successfully as my husband Alan's business manager; but looking at that long term, we both decided that I was denying myself my own creative development and skill base. Then I had focused on business building and development for small business owners, but that too, good as it was, wasn't giving me the fulfilment that I craved. I was wandering around in the wilderness of my life looking for 'the thing' that would re-ignite my spark.

I was recognising the need for space and the importance of it. I had always needed space more than anyone else in the family, but, like many things, I had been denying my own needs until I fulfilled those of everyone else, so had let it evaporate. In this time-out I started to carve out this time again and one of the ways was through walking. I had done very little since my return from Spain, but I knew how happy walking in nature made me. It was that simple. I didn't have the energy to walk far but I did start to take regular short walks again. In nature I felt free, I felt there were no expectations.

I was determined to be aware of what was going on in and around me, but although this sounds easy, when you have not been practicing this, it's quite challenging. I tried to stay in the moment, being grateful for the small things. Keen to try anything that might help, I also turned to some alternative therapies, having regular Reiki sessions and trying meditation. And I caught up with a few friends and colleagues with whom I felt at ease.

I also did a couple of client days when asked, but I was very passive, not seeking out work and having a very low profile on social media. When I tried to do too much my head would hurt, there was literally no space in there for much, so I would stop again. I know now how important it was just to take time out and to do little and ensure that whatever you do is something that brings you joy.

"[Walking] is the perfect way of moving if you want to see into the life of things. It is the one way of freedom. If you go to a place on anything but your own feet you are taken there too fast, and miss a thousand delicate joys that were waiting for you by the wayside."

— Elizabeth von Arnim

Chapter 3

The months went by, I got stronger and felt much better, and in early December 2013 I went out to Vancouver with the family to attend the Global Speakers Summit. It was so good to see my international friends, and one of my favourite places to walk is in Vancouver. Stanley Park is a 405-hectare public park on the edge of downtown and it was very close to our hotel. It offers wonderful woodland, lakes, open space and is mostly surrounded by water. I have walked there often when attending conferences and courses, so even away on business I had this great space to continue my walking. It felt like I was being 'looked after'.

At the conference I was running a break-out session on Virtual Book Tours. Yes, that very thing I had been working on, the one that ended up being the catalyst for discovering my burnout. I had applied to run this session long before my burnout discovery, and as the time came to run it, I was feeling energised and much calmer and happier again.

As most speakers have books, I wanted to share what I had discovered through my experiment with Alan's book. It went very well, there was standing room only and lots of engagement. People loved the concept and at the end so many came up and asked me if I would do this for them. I was ecstatic, clearly this was what I'd been waiting for. This was the new business. This was the thing that I had been looking for. This is what I was meant to be doing. I was so excited, and it felt in a way that the pain I had been through was all to get me to this point.

Once home, I followed up with interested people and then in January I jumped in. I had a clear vision of how it would unfold. Everything started to take off very quickly and I secured clients. I knew the structure I wanted to develop, the team I would need to build and my role. It was all falling into place.

What made it so interesting was the variety of different stories that these people were telling through their books. There were personal stories, many of which were so traumatic that I was in awe of the strength and survival capacity of these authors. There were business books on all different aspects of that world, and some adventure type books, too – again, personal stories but exploring and discovering. I felt really honoured to be working with these people and helping them get their stories out into the world.

For the first eight months all was well. As I was working, I was writing the manual, which is so much easier to do as you go along rather than retrospectively years ahead. I developed a new website and I started speaking more, throwing myself back into the Professional Speaking Association (PSA) and travelling to many of the regions to talk about this

Virtual book tour. There were always lots of interested people and potential clients.

Then, in August 2014, it all came crashing down…again.

We had been burgled in June of that year and, amongst other things, my daughter and I had had our laptops stolen. In August they were replaced, but when I went to restore the information, the back-ups were corrupt. I had lost everything from this new business. It was like someone had punched me in the stomach and knocked the wind out of me. I was bereft. Here I was with a growing business and all the information, details, newly written manual had gone. I felt no one really understood the seriousness of this, and I remember getting really frustrated at my husband who felt that it would all be ok, I would be able to gather all the material again.

I felt the stress return. I was really edgy, and not in good way. My head was feeling so full it felt ready to explode and suddenly there was no space to think or to process. I could feel myself falling back into irritability, frustration and overwhelm, as well as being quick to feel angry. I didn't seem able to explain fully how I felt any more and it didn't seem to be a big issue for anyone else but me. Why did no one else get how awful this was?

I kept going as best I could, serving my clients, and I do know that I can be a great actress, putting on that mask again and giving my performance. I may not have been my usual totally upbeat self in their eyes, but everything was ok. Who was I trying to kid?

Deep down I recognised that I was back where I was almost a year before, not quite as bad, but stressed, overwhelmed, lost and feeling hopeless.

With hindsight, I know that all that was meant to happen. The loss of all the material was because the Virtual Book Tours, although a good business, wasn't what I am here for. I can see it so clearly now, and I am very grateful. But back in September 2014 my desperate thoughts asked, 'Where am I going to go now?'

I felt that black cloud descend once more and there seemed no point in anything. I shared what was happening on Facebook and a couple of lovely friends said, 'let's get together'. On 5th September I met the first, a fellow coach and friend, in the Corinthia Hotel in London. It's the kind of place you get dressed up for, and yet here I was sitting in this beautiful atrium while people around me enjoyed afternoon tea and I was trying to stop the tears flowing and worrying about my mascara leaving streaks down my face. Dion questioned me further in a very kind and caring way and mentioned how 'in my head' I was, and then she said, 'Heather, your body is yelling at you to stop'. 'I know', I answered, 'but I can't'. How ridiculous is that?

I knew how crazy it sounded as I said it, but it felt so true. I couldn't. I mean, what about my clients? What would I do about them? I had made promises. There were expectations!

How many of you identify with that? The feeling that, for your own benefit you have to change things and stop, but as a woman with responsibilities you must be there for others first. I see it all the time.

Through the deluge of tears and the pain that was in me, I kept insisting that I had to fulfil my commitment. I couldn't see any other way. So, we came up with a small plan. I would continue to work with the two clients that were deep into planning their book tours; I would continue organising all the steps; I would use my VA as much as I could; and then when they were finished in a few months I could step back. In the meantime, I would put all other work on hold.

Within a few days of trying to move forward with the plan, I knew that even working with these two clients was too much. I had such little energy and interest that I just couldn't tend to them. When I tried to think my head would hurt, everything took so long, and technology and I were as far apart as we could ever be. I had to bring a stop to this. I had to stop otherwise I was going to get really sick. I was terrified that I would get so ill, even that I would die, and it would all be because I was not looking after me.

I wanted to speak to my clients in person, but I knew that I would burst into tears and would be unable to say what I wanted to say. I was feeling so guilty about letting them down. The only way was by email, so I plucked up courage and started to compose. I was transparent, apologising for this form of communication and explaining that I would rather be calling them but if I did that I would be in tears. I was totally in my truth and sent the emails off.

The responses were caring and full of concern and love and brought more tears. They could not have been kinder and more understanding. 'Health is everything, you sort that first and then we can speak again', was the message from both. Relief washed through me. Why do we expect the worst scenario? I had been afraid of letting them down and had been concerned how they would see the professional me. By being open, honest and vulnerable, I had given them the true picture, and, as humans, they had given back to me.

This was a lesson that would remain with me.

Stand in your truth, it will never let you down...and it means you can live with yourself, the most important thing.

The second person that offered help was a counsellor friend of mine, and I met her at her home base where I had spent retreat time previously. In this little cabin, warm and cosy beside the wood-burning stove we talked, I cried, and she mentioned the disconnection between heart and head or body and mind. Here it was again, and it jarred for me. This was not me! I always saw myself as someone who was very much in touch with my feelings, too in touch sometimes, ruled by my heart and not my head. I was embarrassed to be seen as someone who didn't have this connection. I was someone who was aligned and connected. My time with Sharon really helped, but I was filled with great sadness as I drove away, questioning what on earth was going on and how was I going to put this right? I wanted to fix it, but I still wasn't sure I could.

A couple of days later, I went to see a cranial sacral therapist. As you might gather, I was searching, searching for the person or thing that could unlock me, unstick me, and perhaps in some deep place, I was hoping for a magic wand even though I knew it didn't exist.

I had never been to a cranial sacral therapist before – the work was very gentle, and I could imagine very relaxing. I did get a little of the calming feeling, but I was too stressed, too wired to appreciate it fully. After the session, I got off the couch and we sat down so Sarah could tell me what she had found, and here it was again: 'Heather there is virtually no body/mind connection, it's just about severed.' I burst into tears. This was such a big thing for me. All those emotions of failing; of not being good enough; of being a fraud; of not being in touch with who I was, or more correctly, who I had become. It kind of rocked my world, but as the same message had come from three people who didn't know each other, within the space of about ten days, I knew I had to pay attention.

Again, I was scared. Health is the most important thing you can have; it's now my top value. I would have said it was always up there, but perhaps I was kidding myself. Without health we have nothing. It was clearly time to take this thing seriously and take 'time out' in a big way.

At the same time as all this was going on, I was working with a Somatic Educator to help with muscle pain, especially in my legs. Over the years, the aches and pains had been developing. However, all the work she was doing with me was having no effect at all, even though it was tried and tested with many of her clients. I just knew that it wasn't her, it was me. She told me my muscles were always on full alert, they never seemed to relax. It was like I was ready to fight or flee at every moment.

She asked me when I'd last had my bloods taken, which I must admit freaked me, and I immediately met her question with an abrupt 'why?' She suggested I have them done anyway 'to rule things out'. Meanwhile, based on her intuition, which was indicating something was missing, she started to explore. The more she explored, the more she uncovered, until we came to a point where adrenal fatigue first raised its head.

GPs don't tend to diagnose this as it is not considered as an accepted medical diagnosis; they are only involved with either end of the scale where the adrenals are concerned. The term 'adrenal fatigue' is used more by alternative therapists such as naturopaths and nutritionists to describe what they consider to be the effects of chronic stress – where the adrenals are overworked, which causes them to stop functioning well and leads to adrenal fatigue.

The adrenal glands are tiny organs above the kidneys that manufacture a variety of hormones your body needs to thrive — including the hormone cortisol, which is released when you feel stress. Signs of these glands being overworked are anxiety, depression, aches in the body, bad sleep problems, gaining weight, and digestive issues, amongst others. I had many of these, and so, as well as seeing the GP and having my bloods tested, I met with a nutritional therapist friend of mine and set in motion a saliva test to measure cortisol levels. The cortisol tests take four individual samples of saliva at various points of the day and then map your cortisol levels over the course of a period of 24 hours. This is because cortisol levels vary dramatically, starting high when we wake up and then tapering off until they reach their lowest point late at night. This usually represents something like an 80% drop, which is perfectly normal. The test is sent in the post and returned in the same way and in my case, the results were sent to my nutritionist.

A few weeks later my blood tests came back and I was told by my GP that everything was fine. I also got my saliva test results, and on the 5 levels of Adrenal Fatigue, where 5 is the worst, I was at 4.

For me it was so liberating to have some diagnosis. I really felt that now I could start to move forward and begin to rebuild my health. The euphoria didn't remain for too long, though, as it was clear that this was not going to be a magic wand rapid recovery. This was going to take time. I knew that the burnout and adrenal fatigue (AF) had been building for years. There was a great deal to undo, a great deal to learn about, and much to put right.

I am concerned, though, as to what would have happened if I had only gone with what my GP said. How long would I have continued in this place I was in, probably blaming myself and believing that somehow, I was the cause of all this. I have plenty of time for doctors and for our amazing NHS (National Health Service), but on this occasion I felt that they were not able to be there for me. With what I know now and what I have experienced, I believe that we have a hidden epidemic of adrenal fatigue. When I meet stressed, overwhelmed, busy women who I feel are probably part of this, I do talk to them about options and alternatives but at the end of the day the choices they make about their health is theirs.

I want to be clear here that this is my story and what happened to me and what I did as a result. If you find yourself in a similar situation you must do what is right for you.

"I love walking because it clears your mind, enriches the soul, takes away stress and opens up your eyes to a whole new world ."

– Claudette Dudley

Chapter 4

I had first worked with Joanna Martin in 2012. In November 2014, after taking time out with her first child, Jo returned with the first One Woman Conference, and with that the introduction to her new business, One of Many. I attended this high-energy, woman-filled event, catching up with so many friends and colleagues and making so many new connections. Here was a tribe that I felt part of – they were speaking my language. There was time and space to look at all that we women were facing, permission to make changes, to connect with our feminine, and approach life and business in a different way.

This all coincided nicely with what I was going through, and I became part of a year-long programme called Lead the Change. It resonated strongly, as in my journey to recovery I was looking at where this stress, this unhappiness and this disassociation were coming from. I was laying out a map of my life on the table and superimposing over it the Wheel of Life tool that I and a lot of coaches use as an aid to exploration. In this way I was able to closely at life under eight headings: friends and family; health; money; career; physical environment; fun and recreation; personal growth; and romance/significant other. The Lead the Change programme modules looking at wealth, love, fulfilment and vitality mirrored this for me. It felt the right thing to do…in both my head and body. Perhaps I was starting to make some progress.

For me, this was take two. My initial burnout in 2013, and then the fact that I hadn't done enough....or taken it seriously enough. Was I really blaming me? Isn't this what we women often do? For me, it was also a sign that all was still not well and that I was not who I wanted to be.

I had stopped working. This was strange – since Saturday jobs as a schoolgirl, I had always worked – but I did understand the need to stop. So often we fill our days with things so that we don't have to look at what's not working. It's rather like sticking your fingers in your ears and going 'la, la, la, la la' or covering your eyes as a child and saying, 'I can't see you so you can't see me'. Sadly, it's not that simple, and I knew that nothing was going to change until I gave myself the time and space I needed. In working with my own clients in the work I do now, it's time and space I am often giving them because I know how important and necessary it is.

I was spending my time feeding my body with good food. So often we miss the difference that good nutrition can make and I, a bit of an all or nothing girl, can go through phases of eating really well and then letting my sugar cravings run wild and my love for bread take over. I bought a Nutribullet and started to make great smoothies and got the juicer back out of the cupboard. I felt that meditation could help, so I enrolled in a 21-day meditation programme and I started to see a counsellor weekly and work with a naturopath. I was determined to recover.

The big issue for me and many others in my position is the amount of money all this costs. None of the above comes on the NHS; there are few, if any, referrals to alternative practitioners and this is, of course, what hampers many getting the help they need. I really appreciate how lucky I was in having a partner who, although self-employed, was making money and was totally supportive of me. Many others are not in this position. Over the next year I was to spend a small fortune, none of which I regret, on supplements, classes, books and courses, as I took responsibility for my own health. How do others less fortunate than me cope?

There are things I did, however, that were free, with walking being my constant. It made my heart sing. Even in this wintertime, I was getting out and walking, often on my own, which was providing me with space and time to think. I found myself using the recording facility on my phone to capture thoughts as I walked. This was also the place I allowed the tears to fall when I felt that the recovery was not quick enough or when I felt misunderstood.

I also walked with the family, too, short forays into Epping Forest and along the river path and usually with somewhere cosy for coffee, hot chocolate or a glass of wine en route or at the end. All these things I loved, and walking was making me more appreciative too.

In January, 'Lead the Change' started. All modules took place as weekend retreats, the first, 'Be Wealth', happened later in the month in a beautiful hotel in the Cotswolds. I have to say that I probably wasn't in my most confident state; I am sure I wasn't the only one feeling nervous. The thought of sharing a room was making me nervous for various reasons, one being that I wasn't sleeping well, and drinking as much water as I drink means I always get up to go to the loo at least once in the night. I had spoken to my roomy as she was also my accountability buddy, so at least she wasn't a stranger, but we didn't know each other. However, I was looking forward to escaping and, as I love to drive, I was happy to find a crisp, blue sky and sunshine day as I left London and headed off.

There was the option of arriving on the Thursday evening for an informal get-together – for setting the scene, allowing folk to ease in and share where they were with regard to the subject matter and, of course, to relax in the knowledge that we were already in situ. I soon felt more at ease. I didn't know anyone except one of the leaders who had been my coach years before when I was starting out, but everyone seemed to be lovely and I could see there were others who were much more out of their comfort zone then I was.

The weekend went well, it was full-on, we covered so much, but I started to make good connections. We walked in the mornings in and around the grounds of the hotel and in the winter crispness our misty breath made me feel alive. We were out for about 30–40 minutes and then back for breakfast, before showering and getting ready for the day ahead. The walks made me feel at home as I didn't have to miss that regular movement that was part of my everyday routine and I had new things to see and to discover. I would have tried to carve out time for this anyway, but it was so much easier it being laid on, and walking with others, especially new people, is a great way to get to know them.

We also danced, led by Susie, and I let my body feel into the music. I used to love to dance and move to music and, although I felt very conscious in the beginning (I think most of us did), I soon learnt to let go and not to care about what others might think. We had done some of this at the conference, and this form of dancing (more like 5 Rhythms) was not about necessarily dancing with anyone else but letting your body embrace the rhythm and music and flow. It reminded me just how important this was to me; it was definitely playing a part in mending that body/mind connection. I came away from the weekend retreat feeling 'I can handle this', as well as with a notebook full of tasks to implement.

There was a project involved with the Lead the Change programme, but I felt that this was something I just wouldn't be able to cope with. Although recovering, I was so scared of finding myself back in that horrible place again, taking on too much, that I was constantly monitoring what I was dealing with. After all, this was me taking time out to focus on me; I just didn't need to put myself under any pressure. The support was there, and I was given the opportunity of making myself the project – my recovery, my self-care and my transition into a life free of burnout and adrenal fatigue when that time came. That was something I could definitely do.

As well as the retreats, this programme had twice-monthly Zoom calls, where we reported on progress, bounced ideas about and supported each other. It was also a great way to further build the relationships that had begun at Be Wealth. I really enjoyed being part of my new circle of women, a group with whom I have a very special bond, even today. There were often opportunities to meet up with one of more of the group, and, as we are all spread out all over the country, social media, Zoom calls and the phone make it easy to keep up to date. We have seen each other at our lowest, in floods of tears and battling demons; we have also been able to celebrate together, to pick each other up and to laugh.

I have mentioned my need for and love of time and space, but this can be hard to get when you have a husband and daughter at home. At this point, my daughter was in her last year at school. My time out was good timing in many ways, as I had been able to go university open days and applicant days once she had been offered a place, and to help with applying for her finance. I was hoping that all would go well and that she would leave home. That sounds like a terrible thing to say, but I knew that she needed this for her own growth and development and that it would also be good for Alan and me.

The years from 14–16 had been most challenging in our relationship, and her GCSEs and AS times were especially hard for me, mainly in terms of studying. Ellie is a very bright girl and so could get where she wanted with doing less work than I ever had to do, but as with many parents, I wanted the best for her. The more I pushed, the more she railed up against me and did the opposite. Now that we had got to this A-level stage, I had at least learnt what battles to fight and had backed off, but it still wasn't easy. I had to bite my tongue so many times, and it didn't stop the stress that I was feeling.

On many occasions, I just wanted to escape, to not have to think about anyone else, to not have to make meals, do the washing up, or make beds, etc. Even though I am extremely fortunate to have a husband who shares much in the home, and cooks and shops, I didn't *want* to have to help, or to do what I thought I should do. I love the sea in all weathers so that was where I was looking to escape to; but I wasn't earning, and it did feel a bit of an expense, so instead I planned a couple of simple day trips. Not quite the same thing, but it helped. And I really enjoyed when Alan was away on business, and he was away a lot at this time. I saw it as the gift it was, and as Ellie tended to stay in her room at this stage, I didn't have to communicate that much. Things were improving in my head generally, but there still felt so far to go. I wanted to be able to click my fingers and have it all sorted.

April brought the second Lead the Change retreat – this one 'Be Love'. I'm not sure which retreat I thought would be the biggest challenge for me, perhaps 'Be Wealth', but it definitely wasn't going to be this one. I was good on love. I had lots of love to share. I had always been someone who shared love, who wasn't afraid to express love.

Why is it when you think that all is going well and in the right direction that everything turns on its head and you realise that this is actually the worst place yet. What happened next showed me that all was far from great – the words 'rock bottom' came to mind.

I had begun to feel this programme was not right for me. I started to become very resistant to what was going on. I thought about it on and off and then about a week before 'Be Love' I sent an email for Jo's attention saying that I wanted to leave the programme, that it wasn't working for me, etc. I think I sent the email on the Friday and on the Monday got a phone call from one of the team. I remember being resistant to sharing anything, very unlike me. I kept saying that I just couldn't continue and that I couldn't come to the retreat. The lovely women I was speaking to pointed out that I couldn't just leave the programme now, that the time for pulling out had passed and I wouldn't get my money back. I, of course, knew this to be true and understood, but I still hoped there might be a way. I shared the situation and then immediately regretted opening up. She suggested that coming would probably do me good, but I kept pushing back and, in the end up, she explained that if it really was not going to be possible, I could carry this through to the following year. Then, of course, it hit me – if I did that then I would be in a different cohort and that would not be as good, even if the women were just as wonderful. Looking at all this from a detached perspective, I was behaving erratically and rather childlike. I left the call saying that I would think about things. I felt so vulnerable and really wished I had stayed quiet.

Later that day, I had a call with my coach on the programme and we discussed the situation. I finally relented and said, well perhaps I would come but if I did, I was not sharing anything.

What was the fear? Judgement perhaps, or the fact that people would see me as weak and perhaps unprofessional. I felt very vulnerable and just wanted to hide. I guess I am not often in this position and, being alien to me, it was so uncomfortable. A few hours later, I phoned the office back and said I would be there.

I made my way to the Cotswolds and felt very uneasy entering the dimly lit room for the evening session. We split into two groups and when they asked for someone to be the one to start, I found myself utter 'I guess I'll start. I've talked about all of this for a few days now I might as well share it all with you too.' I surprised myself. I'd more or less been dragged to this retreat kicking and screaming, and now that I was here, I was stepping up and being visible. The support was amazing and even though the tears were threatening, I didn't feel judged or thought of as less than. I just felt loved and appreciated.

I had booked a room on my own for this retreat. It cost more, and money was something that wasn't at all plentiful at present, but I needed to be able to roam around, put the light on at 3.00 in the morning if that's when I was tossing and turning, and just have the space and peace of being alone. I didn't need to have to worry about anyone else.

The next morning Jo, who of course knew exactly what was happening, came up and gave me a hug and told me she had been waiting for me to have a bit of a meltdown and breakthrough. 'Perhaps tonight', she said.... No pressure there, then?

On the Friday night, Annie was to lead a meditation session, and we were told to come with a towel to scream into and a pillow to thump. We dutifully turned up, and as we all found our self-space in this barely lit room, the crew took their places around the room, there to support in whatever way they could. Jo had taken up a place close to me. I knew she was there to be there for me, but I felt such great pressure to have a breakthrough, to perform in some way. I know that wasn't the intention but it's how it felt.

The session started, and before long the sound of tears and sobbing started from some quarters. I was aware that some of the women were pummelling their pillows and others rocking backwards and forwards. This was a bit of an alien experience for me and I knew that if it all felt a little weird to me that there would be others who might be a little freaked out – this would be totally out of their comfort zone. Nothing was happening to me. I didn't feel any different, I wasn't tearful – 'comparisonitis' was living and breathing. What was meant to happen?

Annie, who was running the session said, 'if you are still seated then get up. Try something different.' I hauled myself to my feet, trying to keep my eyes closed but also keen to peek and see what was going on. I started to sway with the music, Susie's dance sessions returned to me and I just let myself go, taking up more space bit by bit, feeling into the space around me. I was stretching and squatting and turning and it felt really good. I felt a little tearful, but no floods, no sobbing.

When the session came to an end, I was exhausted and headed to bed. Did I do it right? I don't think I did. Why was I so quick to blame or to question myself? Was there a right way anyhow? I think this was all part of the place I was in and had been in, that place where I so doubted and questioned myself. Some things were shifting, but this wasn't, or at least I had yet to see it.

Something did happen, though, because after my shower the following morning, I lifted my eyes to the mirror and for the first time in years I did not recoil from what I saw. I know that sounds extreme, but I had got to the stage of hating my body so much. I spoke to myself in horrible ways. I called myself fat and wobbly and wondered how anyone could love me . Yet this morning, although I did not love everything I saw, I could look. I could appreciate some of the bits of it. I could appreciate this body that had carried my daughter, had given birth to her and fed her. I could start to appreciate some of the curves as well as the fact that my strong legs had carried me on hundreds of miles of footpaths. Yes, I still wanted to be stones lighter, but I was looking at me.

I still can look at me. I can now walk around at home with no clothes on. I can walk around a shared bedroom on retreats and similar in my underwear. This was huge for me, and it was, of course, the first thing I shared with Annie when we met for the first session. She wasn't surprised. She had seen the difference in me when I got up and started to move, she had seen fluidity appear and a softening that went with it. And…there was no right or wrong.

The retreat that I thought would be an easy one for me was the hardest, it was the one that kicked ass, it was the one that dove deeper and brought about a huge realisation. While I may easily and happily show my love for others, the one person I wasn't showing love for was me.

How can others love you if you don't love yourself?

I am still on that self-love journey, because, although I do love me so much more, I am sometimes still pretty horrible to me. Not for those long periods anymore, and not so vociferously, but I still do it when I am in low mode. Then I remember to dance and shake it out or walk, and the fog lifts.

For me, my image is such a pivotal point. Is that vain? Some may say it is. I know that loving yourself internally is more important? But looking good on the outside is important as well, and the external can help to start the work on the internal too. There is not only one way. In this shift, a lot was about external image, and accepting me externally did help me get more to grips with the internal and, in time, vice versa.

When I overeat and eat the wrong things, I feel 'yeuchy', which affects how I feel initially on the inside and then how I see myself externally. It's all tied up. At times like this, I see myself as never being able to lose weight, never being the fit and toned woman I want to be – but that's not necessarily true, that's just my perspective. That's when my language is negative, blaming and shaming, and when I am quick to spark at others. It is me I am annoyed and angry at, but I'm not always able to admit that, so I take it out on others – and those others are my nearest and dearest. Although I could see the reasons for eating more – such as being fed up, disappointed or bored – I wasn't acknowledging the process and how I was, in fact, inflaming things. Because, when I eat well, I feel lighter, my clothes loosen a little and I perhaps lose a little weight, I feel so much better, and then anything becomes possible.

The realisation around my eating patterns and how they made me feel, as well as the impact on others, made me want to shift the weight even more. I kept joining programmes and buying new diet books, but nothing was helping. It wasn't until I learnt about cortisol levels that I realised that all the money and all the diets in the world weren't going to make any difference until I got my cortisol levels down – and that would only happen once the stress was reduced and under control.

This hatred of my body and general hatred of me was not having a positive effect on my relationship with my husband. I didn't want him to see this 'horrible' body, so there was little room for intimacy. I'd grown up in the times of communal changing rooms, had gone to The Sanctuary in central London with girlfriends where we took great delight, with many others, of swimming naked and being in the jacuzzi, steam room and sauna naked too. Now I would hide away.

It's a good job that sex wasn't the key part of our relationship, and I do believe that we weathered this challenging time because we respect and love each other so much. At this time, I finally found the right naturopath to work with, and the alignment of this happening just after the realisation through 'Be Love' was not wasted on me.

Through my walking, I was becoming so much more aware. More aware of what was happening around me as I walked. More aware of what there was to see, and much more aware of how I was feeling. It was slowing me down. I was more grounded. I was more in the moment more often. I felt that that body and mind connection was starting to grow through this simple activity that I loved.

One of the hardest things for me was having to admit that the two people whom I loved most in the whole world were the two people who were stressing me out the most. I held off saying that for so long, except in my head, because I felt I would be betraying them, but once I had articulated it to someone else it was like I was able to see a way to fix it.

I had been in a place where the least little thing would end in a blow-up and me in floods of tears. I would have got to a point where I felt that I was so bad at explaining things that the conversations that seemed to be repeated over and over were happening again, and what was the point. I would become tongue-tied and unable to argue my way out. I would be frustrated, and my husband would tell me to stop being so angry. I recall saying 'I'm not angry, I'm just so frustrated because I cannot seem to make myself understood, yet I am taking ownership of my feelings as I believe is the way to do this, and yet my words are not being heard.' One day I just walked out, picking up the car keys on the way, and drove up to my beloved forest with tears streaming down my face. I sat in the car in an empty car park for hours crying, talking it all through in my head, and at times into my Dictaphone, and trying to make sense of it all. I wondered if I was going mad. I hated what I was doing to those I loved.

'I have a right to be angry. I have a right to be heard.' It seemed that when Alan and Ellie didn't want to hear what I had to say, perhaps because I had shone the light on them, that they would speak over me and often just walk away, bringing the conversation to an end. And when I got frustrated, I would often be told to 'calm down'. That to me is like a red rag to a bull, it incensed me. In the counselling I was attending, we worked on that, tracing it back to my authoritarian dad who believed that we – my mum, sister and I – should share his beliefs and not question. In our house when I was growing up, lively debate and discussion didn't happen. I never really learnt to debate until I did an Open University degree in my thirties, and I am still not that practiced at it. I did, however, make sure that our daughter Ellie was encouraged to ask questions and to have an opinion. I have a feeling that many women of my generation may find themselves sharing some of these experiences. Having a voice is so important, not just for me but for everyone; as I said earlier, I believe it is a right.

In mid-May 2015, I attended a day with Joanna Martin and five of my Lead the Change colleagues. The shift at 'Be Love' was one of the major realisations in my recovery, and I was starting to consider my return to work and how that might look. I was aware that I wanted a gentle re-entry. A lot of growth had taken place for me, a lot of changes had been made, and it was one thing to implement and maintain these when I had very few deadlines to meet and was not working. Much as I wanted to return to being a fully functioning business woman, I was very aware that continuing to work on my recovery and get back to my own business could potentially bring more stressful and pressurised situations when maintenance would not be so easy. This day provided a great opportunity to plan for this.

There are two things that stick out for me on that day. One was the feedback from the others, including Jo, when I pitched the idea of returning to the Virtual Book Tour Business, which would bring in the income while I let the business of taking women walking on the Camino grow organically. The response was unanimous – everyone thought both businesses a good idea, but the passion that came across for the walking business was so much stronger. Jo's words were the ones that mapped out the path ahead. 'In all the time that I have known you, Heather, you have wanted to take women walking. So why don't you stop trying to build a business doing everything else and just do this. Do what you love.' Simple – and deep down I knew it – but I needed this permission. I remember leaving that day feeling so much lighter than I had felt for a long, long time, and feeling happy too.

The other thing that sticks with me stemmed from an exercise in which we had to imagine walking in a forest and a wild animal approaching us. In my visualisation, this wild animal was a deer and I was able to pet it, to stroke it and put my arm round its neck. In the real world that would never have happened. My take on it was that sometimes you have to step back from reality and pursue the dream. I had been putting forward all these reasons why the walking wouldn't happen, but by taking a step back and believing in what I could offer, it did indeed happen – and is still evolving today.

On my way home that evening, I took my favourite road up through Epping Forest via High Beech. It was dusk and I was loving the light and the trees and feeling very contented. As I turned one of the corners, moving off the road into the trees was not one, or even two, but three deer. They stopped and just gazed at me. I shivered. I felt very at peace, and I still get goosebumps when I tell that story or read the account. If I wanted a sign that the decision I had made was the right one, this was it.

In the summer of 2015 I redid my saliva test. I was feeling so much more chilled, I no longer leapt to anger and frustration, and I was definitely making more time for me. Putting myself first had been so hard initially, but now that was coming more easily. I am not sure it will ever be really easy, but I was getting there. The test showed that I was no longer 'adrenally fatigued'! Wow! Although I'd hoped for this result, I don't think I had really allowed myself to believe that I had reached this point. I was initially thrown, but then allowed myself to believe it was true. Did I celebrate? Not in a huge way. I told those I was close to, of course, but it was a while before I shared it widely. I think I was a little scared that I might regress.

There was now nothing to stop me going back to work. My time out had come to an end and, as I mentioned earlier, I needed to move forward a different person. I couldn't return to the me I was before, living my life as I had before. The push, push and the always striving had to change. That's the masculine way, but it was not the way that was going to work for me. It actually doesn't work for the majority of women.

We women are much better at consulting and at collaboration. In the world of work the model is very much the male way. Think about it – the world of work was, in the past, a mainly male domain. Men made the rules and set the processes, and, at that point, women usually worked in support, never in leadership roles. Then as time moved on, there were more women in the workplace, still not in lead roles, but when they got married, they often had to leave, and then definitely when they had kids. It's only in more recent times that women have been in leadership and in positions to have their voices heard, but we still have this masculine role model.

What we need is a different model, one that brings both energies to play because we need a mix of both. There is not a right and wrong; the best is a coming together of both energies and both approaches.

I believe that this masculine energy and approach and the fact that there is often no choice in the workplace but to work in this way, is why so many women burn out. I was a case in point, and the interesting thing for me is that, even when I stepped out and set up my own business, I took this way of working with me. I have seen many other small business owners do the same thing. They left corporate jobs after having children or after redundancy or burnout and set up their own business for flexibility but, especially when having kids and being there for them, they were the women sending emails at midnight or even in the early hours, as this is when they could fit it in. And it wasn't that this is when they worked best and they could sleep in in the morning; no, they would be up for the children or for meetings that were already in their diaries. They ended up working even more hours and putting even more pressure on themselves. No wonder many burnt out.

So, I needed to move forward with a different approach. I had begun to think about this in my day with Jo, but to be honest, that had just skimmed the surface. It had given me the permission and the clarity to pursue my passion, but there was a long way to go yet to make it a reality, and I was still so tied up in this fear of a backward step that I knew I needed to move forward slowly.

One of the great things about my time out had been the opportunity to be there for Ellie in her final year at school. As parents, Alan and I had both attended open days for university, but I had then had the time to return with Ellie to attend 'applicant days'. These were the universities wooing potential students further, inviting them to take part in workshops, etc., in the hope that they would get a deeper flavour of that university and choose it.

It was fun going to these, good mum-and-daughter time, and I felt that being 'full-time mum' for a while longer would be good. It would enable me to get Ellie through the summer and results and then settled into university, and for me to cope with her no longer being at home. We had always prepared Ellie to move away, knowing that university was about more than just the educational side, and that in living away from home she would learn more about herself. I was looking forward to it being Alan and me again, but I wasn't sure how I would feel when it came to the actual time.

All was well, the decisions were made, the results were favourable, so many celebrations took place and in mid-September we moved our only daughter into halls at Reading University. The tears did not flow as I was concerned they would; yes, I was a little emotional, but as we drove past as we left, there was a young woman already in a group of four others chatting and laughing and giving us a brief wave as we headed home. She would be fine and so would I.

An early-morning walk is a blessing
for the whole day.

- Henry David Thoreau

THE PRESENT

Chapter 5

On 5th October 2015, I returned to work, fully recovered from burnout and adrenal fatigue. What I do now, and as a result of what I experienced, is run the business I love. This is one that honours my values. It is part of my chosen lifestyle, one that I have carefully crafted and created. I worked hard to make it so – it didn't just 'appear' – and it takes ongoing work to keep it as I wish it to be. I'm not sure, however, that it would ever have materialised had it not been for the 'gift' of my burnout.

When I tentatively took those first steps back in, I felt myself renewed. I had my spark again and my eyes were shining – that's always when I know whether things are good or not. Eyes truly are the window to my soul, because when my eyes are dull and lifeless, I am, too, and for the last few years there had been a lot of that.

I speak to so many women who are overwhelmed, juggling so many aspects of life; they are busy most of every day and they are stressed with everything life throws at them. I can see in them, and hear in their conversations, so much of the woman I was. The talk is about feelings around overwhelm, busyness, detachment, carrying everyone else, loss of self, and the fact that they have no time for themselves. They use the phrases and words that I, too, have used, and there is likely so much more in layers underneath that isn't even coming out. Their 'mask' is in place. There are some things it's ok to articulate and so much more that we are fearful of sharing. So many women worry that they are 'less than' or 'not worthy'. We are concerned about being seen as weak and not coping. Yes, I had been there.

I am sure that many of these wonderful women are at one of the Adrenal Fatigue levels, and I know where this can lead if they take no action. However, it's not necessarily a case of having to take 9–12 months off, as I did. It's about starting to listen to your body and starting to take some action now. It's nipping this in the bud and not allowing it to develop any further. It's bringing in short periods of self-care, integrating a walk into your day, and starting to look at who you really are. Not the you that others expect you to be. Not the you that society suggests, but the authentic real you. Because when you know that and stand in that truth, everything else flows.

So many women are leading superficial lives, not because they choose to, but because they have no time to dig any deeper. When did you last read a book that wasn't a novel and actually think about what it's saying? When did you last pick up a self-help book and when you got to the exercises, complete them? They take time. So often we say we'll come back to them later, but we don't; or we stop because we are afraid of what we might uncover, or that we won't know how to address it or what to do with it.

Cast your mind back to when you were a young woman. How was the world looking for you? What were your dreams, hopes and aspirations?

At that point in life, the world is our oyster and we are going to reach out and grab it. I know I did. In fact, that stayed with me for many years. But there comes a point when things start to hamper our plans. Jobs and careers have a way of clouding things, so we start to think that perhaps the time to go travelling is not now; better to get established in a career or get that first job and your feet under the table. Then add property. Even renting a place that you grow to love means it's harder to jack it in and reach for something else. And what if you are buying? That's a big financial commitment that comes with the need to make choices. Then partners appear in our lives, which means compromising. Sadly, for some women, they even lose their voice at this stage! Has this happened to you?

As the years pass, children enter the mix for some; promotions and job changes take more time and energy; general happenings, including those we don't want in our lives at all, like ill health, redundancy, etc; we face empty nests as our young people go to university, go travelling or just move out; and then, especially for women, we may have to take on the burden of ageing parents.

As a result of all or some of these happenings, you can arrive at a point later in life where, just like me, you have lost the zest and the very essence of the women you were. It can be a scary place to find yourself in.

As I have said, there was one point in my journey where I wondered if I would ever find my way back to the 'spark' that was the woman I loved to be. The great news is that I did find her again and my eyes sparkle once more, my energy has returned, and, on most occasions, I have a spring in my step and a smile on my face. If you are wondering who you are, or have lost that vibrant, life-loving woman, I am here to tell you that it is indeed possible to rediscover her, to reconnect with her, and to totally re-ignite that spark....and to be an even better version of that woman than you were.

Having been through what I have been through, I have great insight. I know that for years I had not paid attention to the many signs; I had not listened to the voices trying to help; I had pushed back, always believing that when I got things done, when I caught up, that then I would deal with these things. I would bet that many of you have been there too. But the time never comes, because other things will always step in to fill any space created and they, too, need attention. And that is the reality; we need to acknowledge this, because deep inside we know. And then we need to start to change our behaviour and take this seriously – because serious is what it is.

We women are our own worst enemies. As the natural nurturers, we cannot stop ourselves being of help to anyone who needs it. Children, partners, ageing parents, friends, colleagues, our careers or our business – and at the end of that list comes 'us'. Is it any surprise that we never get to us. I liken 'us' to the crumbs that get swept off the table that no one really misses, small and insignificant, and that's what we do to ourselves.

I know we are so afraid of letting others down, which was my thinking in the first part of this book. But, by paying attention to our needs, by meeting our needs (and sometimes that doesn't take long, especially if we are continually doing it), we are in fact in a much better place to help others.

When we look after ourselves first, we are fulfilled and less likely to be resentful and therefore able to give even more.

I wanted to be able to help women who were going through what I went through, and I hoped that I could find a way to nip things in the bud and not let them reach the point that I had. I wanted to stop the burnout happening. I wanted to catch the adrenal fatigue at an early stage so it wouldn't progress.

And I had many ideas of what my role could be in effecting all of this.

*"If you seek creative ideas go walking.
Angels whisper to a (wo)man when (s)he goes for
a walk."*

— Raymond I. Myers

Chapter 6

From my own experiences, I knew the difference walking had brought to me; I knew that through this simple activity I could impact so many others. But perhaps my audience were not yet in the same place as me.

In 2006, when I had first embraced the idea of walking as part of my business, very few people talked about it as a form of exercise or gave it any real credit for its role in health and wellbeing. In late 2006, as a result of training twenty women to take part in a 38-mile trek in aid of breast cancer, I had set up my first walking group and started to explore 'netwalking' events for women in my locality. I had started to take some of my female small business owner clients 'walking and talking' and started a programme to train others to get fit for charity treks. I used my own experience here, from when I had put together a programme of training for myself and a friend, firstly, when participating on a charity walk along parts of the Great Wall of China in autumn 1999 and secondly, when training a small group of women who were doing the Inca trail. I knew it worked.

Now in late 2015/early 2016 the image of walking was changing. It was something now embraced by people of a range of ages; there was much more choice in the gear available, and walking holidays were something friends and colleagues talked about. However, there was still a long way to go to convince others of the power that this simple and easy to do activity had.

I knew that if I could introduce walking to more women, they would start to see the possibilities and the transformations that could happen. I also had the hindsight of knowing what had worked and what hadn't....and why.

It was so important for me to walk my talk thoroughly, and so my day started with a walk. I would leave the house around 7.00 not always knowing where I would go, but, if I trusted, the ideal route would unfold.

Through exploration I had a number of walks I could do from my front door and even more that started from a short car ride away. First thing, the walks tended to be 30–40 minutes long, a great way to start the day, and they became my planning time, my meditation, my 'me' time, and my creative time. Although at other times of the day I would walk with others, these walks were for me only. I did what felt right for me and listened to my intuition. I was now doing this rather than ignoring the voices, so I didn't want anything to stop this flow.

Even in the depths of winter, this was such a great way for me to start my day. It cleared my head and set me up for whatever was happening in the day ahead. When it was really cold, I would lay my walking clothes on the radiator at night so I could reach out and pull them on first thing. In this way I could head straight out before I talked myself out of it, and then I could shower on my return. There is something really lovely about being out there as the world is waking up.

This new business thoroughly reflected the major part that walking played in my life. With my very clear vision of walking with women on the Camino de Santiago, I began to plan to lead my first Camino Experience. It would be in spring 2017 with another in the autumn of the same year. That felt like a big step forward and oh, such a good first step.

In mid-October of 2015, I did the last of my retreats as part of Lead the Change programme. It was 'Be Vital', and the one thing that hit me was how much more vital I was now. The woman I had become through everything I had done was a very different person from the one who had started this programme.

While the Camino Experiences were my passion, I had to get more women out walking, and in a way that was simple for all. Every day, in one way or another, this activity impacted my life, and the more I did it the more it happened. The calling I felt, was growing.

At this stage, it would have to be something that women could do from home and in their own time, and I knew that accountability could help greatly. In January, I set up the Walk Challenge encouraging women to pledge to walk either 1000 or 2000 miles in a year. I know that sounds a huge amount but broken down over 12 months it isn't quite so scary; and when it's broken down to weeks, then it's roughly 19 miles a week. With the average person walking around 2 miles a day, a total of 14 miles in a week is not that far off and if you are joining a challenge, then aren't you motivated to do a little more? For me, 2000 miles in the 12 months was my goal. I wanted to get back to fitness for my Camino Experiences in 2017 and this was a great way to do it.

Very soon I was getting comments like this –

"Getting quite into this walking lark. Walked from Holborn to the National Gallery, then a few times round the National Gallery, must be a few thousand steps there. Thanks to Heather's challenge!"

"My mindset has changed for the better. I really notice the difference when I don't walk as then I seem to fall back into old habits of stressing over silly things."

"I walk as much as I can, am tracking 250 steps every hour for 14 hours a day

and am often found marching up and down the corridor on my hands-free when on conference calls to ensure I meet my target. I walk at lunchtimes even if just round the block but am trying to walk by the canal as the water is so lovely to be beside! I even went out for 30 minutes after dinner tonight as I hadn't quite made my target as it was mostly a day to do chores round the house."

Bit by bit the changes started to become apparent in the women joining, in both small and large ways.

In April, I launched WomenWalking:WomenTalking as a Friday walk initiative. One of my aims regarding halting burnout and adrenal fatigue, was to get women into the way of giving to themselves more. By running a walk once a month on a Friday, my message was: 'Give yourself the gift of a day once a month, get out into the fresh air and walk. It's a chance to discover different parts of London and its surroundings, to laugh and chat, to exercise without it being onerous – and there is always the opportunity to talk business with fellow business owners too.'

These continued into 2017, when I made the decision to do only the Christmas one. We had regularly had a core of 4–6 women, but numbers started to fall. It wasn't that women didn't want to come, but I was regularly hearing, 'I want to come, but I really should finish this piece of work before the weekend'. That word 'should' that so many of us, me included, use regularly (or from time to time). 'Should' is someone else's agenda laced with guilt and sometimes shame. When are we going to learn, that we can choose to set our own agenda and do what we want to do? It's challenging I know, with all the beliefs that we have been brought up on, but we can change it.

Those who didn't come would see the photos afterwards and say, 'It looked like you had such a great walk, I wish I had joined you'. And those who had come would say, 'I am so glad I came, I nearly didn't because of work, but I feel so much better now'. It's a work in progress this mindset-changing, and one I have no intention of giving up on.

The Christmas and Cocktails Friday walk, though, was a very different story. That one is usually oversubscribed, fills early and is one of the highlights of the walking calendar. Is it the cocktails, is it Christmas, or a mix of both? Part of the winding down and part of celebrating, hopefully ourselves, as well as Christmas time.

From walking, I grew more connected with myself and with nature, my surroundings and in turn the natural world and planet. I wanted to bring this to others too because it is a big part of our transformation, our ability to de-stress and to slow the pace. Being mindful and therefore in the moment, especially in nature, has such a beneficial effect on our wholeness. Everyone who wishes to can access the '7 days of Mindful Walking', which is an aid to help those to start discovering this for themselves.

Mindful walking is something we practise on the Camino Experiences and it started to be something that the women would ask for on one-day walks too. Because of practising mindfulness, not always consciously, I am so much more aware of my surroundings as I walk, and this enhances the whole walking experience. I can spot fungi metres away, and I am much more in tune with what is happening throughout the different seasons, not only in the trees and plants themselves, but also looking much deeper at what the seasons could teach us.

Nature is where I head for peace, and calm, for headspace, to be creative, to plan and to let go. In this space, this holistic activity brings me that much-needed connection with body and mind. In my experience being in nature expands our thinking, it clears our head and makes decision-making easier. Through walking, I have time to think and just allow my thoughts to flow. I often say to walking friends and clients that, whether you take your problems for a walk with you so you can walk them through, or leave them at home, you will always find a solution. This is why I choose to use walking for my own health and wellbeing and for my client work.

It's also a great vehicle to use when we need to have challenging and sometimes difficult conversations. When walking side by side, constant eye-contact is not required and it's so much easier to walk through those periods of silence without feeling the need to jump in. I encourage clients to have meetings on foot, and for others to have discussions with partners or family members by taking a walk. Away from our usual surroundings, the combination of quiet and space, the rhythm of walking and the closeness to nature all seem to bring ease and flow to situations.

I used to be the woman who would detox on cold juices and salads in February, wondering why it wasn't working and why I was so miserable. The winter in the northern hemisphere is our hibernation time when many animals will burrow down and go to sleep to conserve energy and escape the cold. Many fatten up to prepare for this time and collect seeds and nuts, etc., to see them through the months ahead if they awaken. Deciduous trees (those that lose their leaves) have their own form of hibernation, called dormancy, that keeps them alive during the winter months. Everything in the tree slows down and there is no or limited cell growth. During this time, the trees conserve what food they have, using it slowly. This is the time of the year, once the leaves have fallen, when you get a great picture of the skeleton branches and shape of the tree. Then, before you even see the first buds in the spring, I always imagine activity happening inside the trees, as they begin to come alive again, and this activity leads to those buds appearing and then the unfolding of the leaves, which gives us hope again.

While it may not be appropriate for us to go to sleep for months on end as animals do, I strongly believe that we can take our lead from nature. Remember, in nature this season is a time of deep stillness, and that, in itself, suggests to me a time to reflect, and to go deep. My personal hibernation begins in December with a slowing down of work, taking time to meet with friends and be with family and to celebrate the year coming to an end.

Moving into January, February, and even early March, is the time when I continue that slower pace. It is my time to be home-based, to build on my plans, to create, to write, to batch material and to take the opportunity to tune into my internal self. It's this time of the year when the weather can be at its worst, and I have found over the years that if I plan too much externally then many things end up having to be cancelled and then rescheduled. I have learnt that I need this quieter time, and I develop a 'hygge' style environment, lighting candles, staying warm, and making nutritious soups and stews. Through all this, I am replenishing my holistic being. I still lead walks and take walks with friends and family, wrapping up well against the elements, and I do my yoga. I am taking care of me and my needs and applying self-care.

Having followed this pattern now for the past few years, I and my business benefit from it, and I enter the next season recharged and excited for what's next.

How can you bring some of these elements of hibernation into your life?

Have a look at your lifestyle and think about what it would mean to take a slower approach at this time of the year. It's one of the things I love to explore with my clients.

Following the cycles of nature is not only about this time of the year, though; it continues through all the seasons. It's about taking the lessons from nature.

Spring is all about growth and renewal. It is the time for new starts and new lives, just look around at what is being born or reborn. For me and my business, this is the time for growth; the time to launch new things; the time when energy is high and momentum accelerates. It's also the time to return to leading my walking experiences and retreats. In fact, some of my annual programmes start at this time of the year. In the countries through which the Camino passes, it's when the weather tends to be warm and pleasant without the oppressive heat and crowds of summer. So late April, May and even early June see me out in France, Spain or Portugal walking and leading groups of wonderful women.

Then, as we head into summer, June and early July is the time for the shorter walking breaks, most likely in the UK. The months of summer are about abundance. The growth continues, and with it the final part of growth, the maturity. Gardens are full of vegetables and flowers and the tree canopies are dense. It's a great time for nurturing relationships, so focusing on family time and shared experiences with friends, but also worth looking at the relationships with colleagues, clients and business partnerships too.

Relaxation, meditation, retreat, nurturing your creative side and rebuilding energy are great things to focus on in this season as the heat can sap energy. Although I love the sun, it's about being aware of the weather and how it affects us and responding accordingly.

Our final season, autumn is about gratitude. This is the time when the harvest is gathered, everything that came to maturity in summer can now be used, and that encourages us to be thankful and count our many blessings. We are blessed by the magnificence of Mother Nature at this time of year as the leaves on the trees change colour. We seem to get some of our best days now – definitely from the walking perspective – often clear and still warm, and this, too, reflects in this being a time for clarity. Again, I am to be found on the Camino. It's also about letting go. The trees are shedding their leaves, what would be right for you to shed? What things can you shake off and then be ready to start anew in the new year?

For many, that back-to-school time can also seem like a new year, and I love this kind of second chance that this is. It's a return to routines, which can help things flow, and in many ways it's a better time to set resolutions or intentions. In my diary, November is the month when I do the main part of my planning and create my strategy for the coming year. A big part of this is reflection on what has happened throughout the past 10–12 months, being grateful for and celebrating all that has been achieved. I take the time to evaluate and decide what needs to be changed, or thrown out, and what new things might appear – and this is in all areas of life. I am preparing for the new year and doing it at this time allows me to 'segway' into the Christmas period smugly, knowing that all is in place to start again in the year ahead. It also allows me to start that process of hibernation, and so the cycle continues.

Scientists at the University of California, Berkeley, in collaboration with UC/Davis, have found that people who practice gratitude consistently report a host of benefits:

- Stronger immune systems and lower blood pressure

- Higher levels of positive emotions

- More joy, optimism, and happiness

- Acting with more generosity and compassion

- Feeling less lonely and isolated

Gratitude leads to having even more to be grateful for, and it's something I try to practise every day. Sometimes it's hard, but at such times even getting to the end of a horrible day is something to be grateful for, as is going to sleep. I find that the turning of the seasons is a great reminder of the wonderful opportunity to review and then to declutter, creating both mental and physical space for whatever will come next.

In early 2016 I had committed to another training, which would start in 2017, and which I knew would greatly support my work with my women. I also started to work with another mentor, Fabienne Frederickson who was at that time based in the States. I had followed Fabienne for a very long time and had seen her grow and develop and fully walk her talk. I loved her honesty and vulnerability and knew that one day I would work with her; so, when she ran a half-day training in London, I seized the moment. I was just going to go and not sign up for anything, but when someone you value talks about how we ask for things and then, when they are in front of us, we say we're not ready and run away, I knew that if I walked away from this I would be doing just that, so I took the leap and signed up. In the afternoon session, I gained so much value that I knew I'd done the right thing…and the timing was perfect. This programme was all about business, and as I started to grow this new business, I had the framework, the support and the recipe to do what I needed to do.

The live events for this programme were in the USA and at my first live event in Florida I sat beside a woman who, when I said what I did, immediately said, 'I have been wanting to do this for so long. I'm coming with you'. I smiled and said, 'let's talk' – inside the butterflies were dancing with excitement. She became my second sign-up for my very first Camino Experience. Since then, she has become a great friend and supporter; she came with me again in 2018 and has committed to at least one more. Through our friendship, Debby has introduced me to other women in her area who love walking, and I have had the pleasure of meeting them and walking with them when I have been visiting. We have connected on social media and I have been able to advise and guide them on walking and some have also joined some of my online programmes. I feel very blessed to have and be developing this following in North America, as walking is a global activity and I have walked in some of the wonderful National and State parks there. Everywhere opportunities for walking adventures of all lengths and for all abilities abound.

During 2016 I was still on my journey of recovery, and I was learning how to live this new life as I stepped further and further into being back in business full-time. Carving out 'me time' was now key. Honouring myself and my values is a priority. Revisiting and reviewing are woven into every month. And it's still easy to slip…. It was, and still is, important for me to be transparent, sharing the good and the not so good, modelling the behaviour I speak about. I talk about stepping back when I know that things are not in flow and why, and gradually more women are paying attention. Being held accountable is also important, so I deliberately put myself into places where I can be held to my actions. My network and mastermind group, as well as a couple of close contacts, are the people I turn to and the people I ask for help. That, however, is still a work in progress.

"All truly great thoughts are conceived by walking."

- Friedrich Nietzsche

Chapter 7

My first Camino Experience took place in May 2017. I had made a conscious decision to do this first Experience in France on one of my favourite sections. In France, the path is quieter, very beautiful and less commercialised. The churches, of all sizes, tend to be open, the food is, as you might expect, excellent, and I knew the women would love the scenery. Our starting point was the beautiful town of Cahors, more specifically, at the 14th-century Valentré Bridge which is an UNESCO heritage site. Crossing the bridge was a great place and way to mark the start of a likely transformation. It also brings with it a great story of the building of this Devil Bridge.

I couldn't have hoped for a better Experience in all senses of the word. Of course, there were things that would need tweaked and changed, but my vision of a small group of women laughing, chatting, walking, pondering and supporting each other was there from the very beginning. The group bonded quickly and, thanks to social media, the friendships that developed over that intensive week are still in place. Through long days, varying terrain and, in some cases, injury, these women walked on and always had time to be joyful and grateful. They left with plans that included issues we had discussed on the path; two even signed up straight away for the following year.

These words are how the women described the experience:

"I loved the group, reaching the tops of hills , the countryside and the challenge. If you are thinking of doing it, do train. The fitter you are the more you will enjoy it." Ros H

"I am so glad I took part in the Camino Experience and really value it. I felt physically good and able to cope though there were challenging sections of steep ups and downs. It was all very positive, well organised and I felt well supported." – Celia C

"Learning so much about myself and how I cope with adversity. Big thanks to Heather for the opportunity and my fellow walkers for the support." – Linda E

"Getting away and completely unplugging for 5 days, being completely open to what the Camino would bring to me, has been nothing short of life altering. It was one of the most rewarding experiences I have ever had, and I've already signed up for the next one." – Debby K

For me there had been difficult decisions to make, one that involved putting one of the women in a taxi to the next hotel so she could rest up after she twisted her knee. My intention of giving everyone an hour's coaching session on the path as we walked was not possible, and I learned that the distance on some of the days was just too long in a group of this size. However, I could see that, generally, the structure was a great one, that all the accommodation and food worked well, and that other personal development tools and mindful walking really enhanced the experience. This is why we trial things and do so from a place of openness and a desire to learn and make it even better.

As with all I do, for me, this is not just about the walking, it's about so much more: the scenery we walk through; the history of the area and of the path; the architecture; the people in the group and those we meet along the way; the food and wine of the season and the locality; and the fact that we are getting to see parts of a country that we probably wouldn't get to see if we were tourists. And then there is what the walking and the experience gives us.

The reason I have designed it this way is that I want the women to have as few distractions and interruptions as possible, so that they can focus on themselves. By deciding to come, they are giving themselves a gift of space and time, so I want to make sure they maximise this for their full benefit. Groups are purposely small, so that we can create a safe environment for sharing, for discussion and debate. And the women are encouraged to walk alone for periods, for the experience itself, but also so they can focus on their thoughts that are coming up. For many, this is not at all easy. When we live busy lives, we fill every moment and then we don't have to address some of the things that may not be working; we can bury our heads in the sand, whether consciously or otherwise. When everything is stripped back and all the things that need doing are done for you, that space and time is there. Much of what we may have been ignoring is right there in front of us. There is no escape. This is why, with my experience, my coaching, my ability to nurture and to hold that space, I love to be able to facilitate their journey and guide them through.

In late September of 2017 I completed my own Camino and finally walked into Santiago. I felt such excitement as I stood on Mont Gozo beside the sculpture of the two pilgrims looking out towards the city, and glimpsed, for the very first time, the spires of the cathedral.

My walking buddy and I had decided not to make the last day a shorter day as many others do, and rush to get to Mass at noon. I had visions of this being a route march, with much of my gaze being on my watch and not enough on enjoying this last section of the journey, which I felt deserved the same reverence as any of the others. It was the right decision, as we had time to enjoy the walk, to stop for the usual coffee and lunch, and to spend some time catching up with others we had met along the way.

Hilariously, we lost our way on Mont Gozo. Signage is not very clear there and we walked around in circles among many empty buildings whose purpose we weren't quite sure of. Finally, we escaped and were more or less immediately into urban walking. Concrete, traffic, roundabouts and the hustle and bustle of a city. On we walked, at this point making our way through the new town with nothing particularly amazing to capture our interest. It was mid-afternoon and, as often happens towards the end, tiredness takes over. It doesn't matter how many miles you have walked, knowing that this is the end means that you cannot envisage even going a mile further and, of course, every mile seems twice if not three times as long as every other. We looked for the cathedral everywhere, but it seemed to have disappeared. 'How can you lose a cathedral of that size'? we asked each other, amazed that there was not one element of it to be seen. We considered a stop for a drink but the only drink we craved was the one at the end.

After negotiating a large junction where many roads came together, we started to head down a hill and the road became narrower. Almost immediately, we were looking in the shop windows of smaller shops, full of ceramics and leather and jewellery. Things were seeming 'older' and at the foot of the hill, once over the crossing, we were into the old town. I could feel the excitement building, it was bubbling up inside me like fizzy water or, more appropriately, champagne. We were walking on cobble stones; the shops were full of Camino symbols and most of the people around us were other pilgrims. We had found the cathedral again and were now just following those ahead, safe in the knowledge that they were heading where we wanted to go.

We entered the square, the Obradoiro Square, by walking down steps and through an archway and then more steps on the left of the cathedral as you look at it. On our way down, who was coming up but the group of lovely Irish people we had met practically every day on this last section and who we had last seen on Mont Gozo as we all took photos. We all hugged and exclaimed our 'well done' wishes, and then there we were.

I am not sure in those first moments that we were really aware of the enormity of what we had achieved. Perhaps it was because we had done this long walk in sections, so this seemed like just another ending of a section not 'the end'. We took photos, of course, and had one taken of the two of us together and stood there looking round and soaking it up. It wasn't until later, when we had our certificate or even the next day, watching others arrive and when attending Mass in the cathedral that we really fully came to terms with having finished that 1000-mile journey started nine years before. I remember when I first started I felt a little of a 'cheat', doing it in sections and also not carrying all my gear and not sleeping in the hostels' but then I met a gentleman who said' 'but you've walked it all, haven't you?' Yes, indeed I had. And then someone else commented how he admired my determination to keep returning to the place I had finished the year before and pick up from there. He said he felt that was so much harder than doing it all in one go. I don't believe that there is a right or wrong way. There are choices, and it is about doing it the way that suits you and creating your own routine and what mileage you choose to cover and how long to take.

I am not religious; I am spiritual. I knew I wanted to attend Mass in the cathedral in Santiago. I knew that from near the beginning. It was an ending for me, it was a chance to say thank you, and it was also to experience the theatre of this moment. By the time we arrived in Santiago, the film 'The Way' had been out for several years, and I tended to watch it either before or after each section. One thing featured in the film, and something that adds to the theatre of the Mass, is the chance of being at the service when the silver incense burner, the 'Botafumeiro', is swung. We hoped that this might happen but were careful not to get too attached to the possibility, and so I really did focus on the moment and the calm and soothing voice of the priest who delivered much of the service. In Spanish there was little I understood but the word 'Peregrino' was mentioned often. I felt really proud to be one of those, one of those 'pilgrims' who had made this journey and taken so much from it. Even during my most challenging years, I had been able to walk.

As mass continued, it became clear that we were blessed as we realised that this ritual with the incense burner was indeed going to take place. It is a sight like no other and when in full swinging mode it seems to be at risk of hitting the cathedral ceiling high above the congregation. The sight was breathtaking for us watching, but what I loved was that, having been told in advance that we shouldn't take any photos, nearly all the priests up at the altar as the Botafumeiro was swinging, took out cameras from their robes and videoed or photographed the event. It brought a smile to my face. These priests were just as fascinated as we were.

I have walked into Obradoiro Square many times since that time and every time is just as special. I feel the magic of the place as I get close and feel the tingles through my body…and in most cases I have the added pleasure of seeing the faces of those I have brought with me who are seeing it for the first time.

On this occasion, the front of the cathedral was covered in scaffolding, as major refurbishment was taking place so that the cathedral is ready for the next Holy Year in 2021. It is a Holy Year on the Camino whenever St. James's Day (25 July) falls on a Sunday. When I was back in spring 2019, the work on the front of the cathedral was complete but the inside was now being worked on so it looked very bare, though those who had come to see the relics of St James could still do so.

How wonderful it will be when all work is complete, and the very special Pilgrim Mass can return to its rightful place.

"Walking . . . is how the body measures itself against the earth."

— Rebecca Solnit, Wanderlust: A History of Walking

Chapter 8

With my clients I use 'Plant Ally' and 'Tree Wisdom' cards designed and illustrated by the talented Lisa McLoughlin. Picking a plant or tree card looks to a meaning of this plant or tree and we use them on the Camino Experiences, as well as on other programmes, to act as a prompt and to be considered during our day or time together. I am always fascinated by the 'uncovering' that results from choosing a card, and I am not immune.

On the autumn/fall Camino Experience in 2017, I as well as all the other women, picked a card to start our day. On this day, we were walking along the Canal du Midi in France, a beautiful and flat path giving us a different journey from the ups and down of the days before. I was pondering my card as we walked. I had picked the Speedwell card and speedwell is about healing. As we walked that day, for most of it on our own – three single women walking at our own pace and with our own thoughts – I pondered the possible messages for me in this card.

In my recovery I had been looking at all elements of me, the emotional, the spiritual and the physical. None is ever completed to a point where you can forget about it, though, as our journey always continues, but I knew that the first two were in a good place. It was the physical health side that I felt still needed a lot more work. I was heavier than I would have liked, my fitness, although pretty good, required more up-levelling and I wanted to bring more flexibility through something like yoga as well. I talked to myself and to the Universe as I walked and asked that, if I was right, the Universe send me a sign – but not a subtle one – so I would know.

For me, white feathers are reassurance and a sign that I am on the right path. When I see them, I always say thank you, but this morning I hadn't seen a white feather at all. All that changed in the next few minutes, white feathers were everywhere. Caught in the tree branches, in the grass along the canal side, even fluttering to the ground in front of me. I had my answer and I smiled in gratitude and in awe at how this works.

Later, at the end of the day as we enjoyed our celebratory drink, I asked if I could share what had happened for me. One of the women asked, 'So what are you going to do to address this, what action are you going to take?' Being pinned down in this way was great – I was not the only one coaching – and I talked about the plans I had considered as I walked. She seemed happy with my response and because I had been asked about this by a client, I felt even more accountability to see it through. On the path, it's also about my learning, my journey, and I love that, although I get to lead and guide, I also get to be part of it and to develop too.

This is why 2018 was very much dedicated to continuing my own physical health journey through a number of steps. Firstly, joining a restorative yoga class, then increasing my 1-2-1 walking and making it the same first thing in the morning priority I had enjoyed previously as well as using the Walk Challenge initiative to get not only the members taking more action, but me too. I threw in some optional mini challenges throughout the year and some photo competitions.

With Christmas and New Year over, one can sink into a bit of gloom, as the weather tends to be cold and damp and getting out is hard, so I launched a 9-day 'Kickstart your Walking' Mini Challenge. Every day for nine days I posted a video of me out there walking; others joined in. Having to take this action and be visible and present to others works well for me and, after that had come to an end, I was back in flow.

I also booked to go and walk the St Cuthbert's Way, a 62-mile path following in the steps of the monk Cuthbert from his base in Melrose in the Scottish borders to Holy Island, also called Lindisfarne, off the North East coast of England. My friend and Virtual Assistant Nicola was going to join me, starting on April 30th. I wanted to challenge myself, and Nicola, who had embraced walking after meeting me and who was experiencing many of its great benefits, wanted to increase her walking too.

The walk was one of the best I have done, its scenery beautiful, and, although I knew the borders of Scotland, this walk took both of us to places never experienced before. I am not sure I would lead a group on the complete walk as it is fairly challenging on the middle two days and the days are long, but the experience of walking over to Lindisfarne and our time spent there was very special. I have it in mind for the first of my UK 3-day walk retreats, with shorter walking days, enabling me to offer more time for reflection, discussion, journaling and exploration.

The St Cuthbert's Way seemed to mark a transition for me food-wise, too, and I came back wanting to review my diet and build on the work I had done with my naturopath. To my delight, this turned out to be relatively easy and the summer months saw me drop a lot of weight, get into yoga flow, treat myself to a week-long MFR (Myofascial Relief Therapy) intensive, and be in the best shape for a long time for both my daughter Ellie's graduation and my 60th birthday. I was fitter, too, and went off in mid-September to walk part of the Camino Frances again from St Jean Pied de Port to Logroño, and then lead a group from Logroño to Burgos. It felt so good to be in such great shape and for everything to be relatively easy. I was even starting my day, while away, with 20 minutes yoga and then doing a day's walking.

Throughout 2018 and 2019, my walking group were walking sections of the North Downs. The South Downs had been our original goal, but access to and from there on a daily basis by public transport is more challenging that we had thought, whereas on the North Downs day trips are easy. On that, we soon realised that the route is also, in many places the same route as the Pilgrims' Way from Winchester. When the long days ended, it therefore seemed a good plan to start the London to Canterbury leg of the Pilgrims' Way, hence this approach. In 2020, we may manage to complete both, unless something more interesting comes up, one never knows.

I love to walk a long-distance path. There is something very satisfying picking up where you left off every month and forging on till the destination is reached. There is also a great feeling of achievement on completion, and the bonus of discovering a whole new area of your own country or someone else's.

My own personal walking exploration and development is very important to me. I have a real need to walk for so many reasons – my personal and professional development, my health and wellbeing, and the fact that it makes me feel so good and keeps me grounded and in touch. Some years allow more exploration that others and wanting to experience another Camino path was important because of my own curiosity and because I wanted to look at some alternatives to offer clients. Therefore, the time was put aside in the diary to walk from Porto to Santiago and to include the little walked Spiritual Variant towards the end, as an alternative between Pontavedra and Padron.

It is indeed a path walked only by a few. Accommodation is limited, but it is very beautiful and the views at many of the high points stunning. Day 2, which brought us along the Ruta da Pedra e da Auga (Route of Stone and Water) was particularly stunning. This is a 7 km route that follows the Armenteira River as it flows down the mountain and consists of 51 mills along the way. We really enjoyed this experience but, although I considered it for clients, there are three long days and it ends in a boat journey, which is wonderful if the weather is good. However, the boat is an inflatable, so it could be horrendous if the weather was bad because you would either get soaked, or should the boat trip be cancelled, it's a long day of walking instead. This is why it is important for me to walk a route for myself before I lead clients.

When I walk, I always learn, be that from clients, walking buddies, or from the time on the path that provides me with the opportunity to think in the same way that it does for my clients. One of my great insights this time was the fact that on the 7th day of a 13-day walk I had a real 'down' day.

It had been a challenging day, a long day, and one that at times was not very inspiring. The end bit was walking into a big city, hardly ever an enjoyable experience and, faced with what seemed like an impossible task of finding our hotel, we took a taxi to get us there. So glad we did, as a fellow pilgrim told us later that it had taken him two hours to find his hotel.

If you had told me that night that I could get the money for the rest of the journey refunded, I would have seriously considered flying home. As it was, all I needed was a good night's sleep and I was back full of energy the next day. I had walked many 6-day sections, and perhaps 7 days once, and this made me so much more aware that for many of my clients, day 3 or 4 of their 5 days is when they might just have their own 'down' day. I am now in an even better position to prepare them for the likelihood of this and support them through it, while reassuring them that this is totally normal.

I cannot reach everyone I want to reach through walking if I am going to walk with them in person. It also limits me to people in my geographical area or only with those who come from further afield on a Camino Experience or similar. The other thing is that I can see the benefits of walking at all levels, so it doesn't have to be long-distance walking or walking that takes you away from home, it can be a walk round the block or to the local park. My aim is to introduce the activity and what it brings as well as the impact it makes, and that can be for anyone at any stage.

The time had come to look at how I could bring walking to even more women worldwide. To meet that wish, I developed an online 30-day programme looking at using walking in small chunks of 10–20 minutes, easy to build into your everyday life, perhaps even more than once. I tested this out for myself along with others on the pilot group working through every step. This is using walking for headspace, meditation, 'time out' and to de-stress – all the things that had helped me, impacting on my mental health in my recovery from burnout and adrenal fatigue.

I then developed a guide to creating walking adventures. The Walking Toolkit which is full of tips and suggestions to make this as easy as possible is available as a downloadable PDF at present, but large enough to become a book in its own right. Of course, like so much of what I develop, it's applicable to women and their friends and family wherever they live.

From a coaching and personal development perspective, I have been trying out possible ways of supporting and enhancing the lives of wonderful women to achieve what allows them to be their true selves in life and live a life that they love. This comes through in the Camino Experiences but also in group and 1-2-1 coaching. This includes online and in-person coaching and nurturing programmes, which are ongoing in their evolution with feedback from clients informing their direction of growth. I so want to be able to bring this to everyone who wants it, whoever and wherever they are. This can be delivered over Zoom and to work with me you don't have to be a passionate walker.

I was delighted to be given the opportunity in 2018 to write a chapter for a book called 'My Camino Walk#1'. It was a compilation of the stories of 19 people who had walked one or more of the Camino paths. I had always felt a book would happen at some time, and I had started a few, but this came at just the right time – funny thing that. I guess everything was in alignment now and I was very proud to have my story included. In writing the chapter, I revisited my memories of this adventure and took time to pull out the impact that it had had on me and continues to have. Writing this encouraged me to see that my own book was a real possibility. Once the doors to making this real opened, the possibility for not only one book followed, and so, as I bring this one to a close, the next book, more of a business approach, has been started. I have also collected ideas and prompts for a series of workbooks possibly linked to a coaching programme.

I have said it before – for me this is all about so much more than just the walking. The walking is the vehicle, it's something to be loved and enjoyed, but walking is also the gateway to transformation and to a long list of mental and physical health benefits. I used to want to be the person who brought the world back to walking, and in the last couple of months that has crystallised further. My wish, and therefore my mission, is to impact the lives of One Million Women through this simple, though often under-rated, activity of walking. For me it's a given that this also includes being in nature as walking often takes us there and once in nature there is so much healing and inspiration to be found.

This took the first step to becoming a reality on 1st November 2019, when I announced my mission and launched a Facebook group called One Million Women Walking. By the end of that first weekend we had 500 members, and this is still growing consistently. We have women from all over the world, and it's a group filled with love and kindness, caring, sharing, support and of so many posts.

Walking: the most ancient exercise and still the best modern exercise.

Carrie Latet

THE FUTURE

Chapter 9

As I stand on the edge of not just a new year but a new decade, I am excited about what is possible. At the end of the next ten years I will be 71, which I find totally unbelievable. In my head I will always be 37! I still intend to be fit and healthy and to be walking with groups of wonderful women, and to still be exploring new walks and bringing new offers to my clients far beyond that age. I intend that many more women will be seeing and also practicing the art of self-care and self-love to themselves every day knowing that they deserve it and I also intend to be still coaching and nurturing my clients as we walk because it is on the path, where I find that the greatest breakthroughs occur. Through this, I love being able to help women find their true selves just as I did and to move forwards clear and unstuck.

I was not in my late twenties, thirties, or even forties when I set up my walking business, and so much of what I am doing moving forward is about legacy and what I leave behind. That suggests times when I am no longer here... The good news is that I have no intentions of leaving for a long time and I have a growing vision, which I know will continue to evolve, and I plan to be right in the middle of making that happen for as long as I can. It's really exciting, if also a little daunting, to be in this place.

Age is not something I think about on a regular basis. I may acknowledge it on a birthday but, after all, it's just a number and not necessarily one that tells an accurate picture. I am sure we have all known people who are much younger and appear older and vice versa. However, it's also a great privilege to have the opportunity to consider what we might leave and what our time on this earth might have meant. I know many of my peers, especially those who have chosen to take control of their destiny, who are doing the same. It's never too late or even too early to think about this.

So, what about you? What might your legacy be?

As a young woman going off to university and escaping from the political situation in Northern Ireland and a life full of bombings, shootings and unrest, I had a vision of how life might look. That included being married by 25 and having the average two children, working as a part-time speech therapist and living in Scotland. Clearly that didn't happen; but lots of other things did, many beyond my wildest dreams. Places I have travelled, people I have met, things that I have got involved in, and these opportunities continue. As far as I am concerned, my age has nothing to do with them, though reflecting a little as I write, perhaps the wisdom of being older and the experience gathered along my journey has made me more open to stepping up and stepping out.

To be honest, there are times when the vision I have is so big that it really scares me and gets me asking 'Who do you think you are to…? This usually happens more so when I start to put the idea into practice, rather than from the vision itself. At the end of the day, the reason I can do so many of these things is because of the support network that I have built around me. Not only family and friends, but often, more importantly in business my colleagues who understand what I might be looking to do.

When I was that young woman, and even in my mid-thirties, I would never have thought that I would have started my own business, nor that at this age I would have no plans to retire. Doing what you love means you tend to want to do even more of it. The fears are still there, though, and the pressures that we find ourselves facing. For me, with such activity in my business, I do find myself thinking occasionally what will happen if I don't look after me? What if I get ill?

Those are questions that are important for us all to consider at all stages of life, and I have given talks where I share the importance of us making health and ourselves a priority. Walking is a big part of my self-care and I know that, for things to look much better, all I have to do is get outside and take that walk. However, even now, years after my recovery, I have to make sure that I don't take my health and wellbeing for granted. It's so easy to slip up, and in busy times especially, let some beneficial practices go. Knowing yourself well, trusting your intuition and being aware, goes a long way to ensuring that you can read the signs and take the required action. And don't forget, that if you ignore these signs your body will step in and make you stop!

My biggest fear and doubt recently, has been around this book. I have started three books over the last number of years and perhaps someday the material written so far will be used. They remain unfinished due to changes in my direction, though that has in some ways come full circle. This one started as part of a challenge. It got so far and then business life stepped in. When I knew that the time was right for this book to see the light of day, I picked up where I'd left off, initially took big strides, and then procrastinated. What if no one wants to read it? What if I can't write? Who am I to write a book?

Sometimes, when I read through it, I think it's quite good; other times not so much. It's fear that often stops us in our tracks, though if I hadn't procrastinated for a while then the One Million Women Walking campaign might not have been included here, as it's so recent, or there would have had to have been a rewrite. Perhaps that was meant to happen? The number of women who tell me that they are looking forward to reading this does make me excited…but what if it's a disappointment?

It's time to stop overthinking, to embrace the moment and to take the leap knowing that my safety net, whatever the outcome, is in place. Getting older doesn't stop the fears and second guessing. And I am sure that when this book project is over there are other major undertakings ready to give me the same challenges, but isn't that what fuels us and keeps us vibrant and connected?

My main piece of work over the next year or two at least is to grow the 'One Million Women Walking' campaign and to see it truly come to life. What we have achieved so far has already been amazing. On that first weekend when 500 women joined, I was astounded and delighted that clearly my wish and intention was resonating with so many other women worldwide. In this time of uncertainty across the world, walking is a constant and provides so much good. This simple activity is a connector. I see it every day through my work and through the group.

Only last week, one of the women from the One Million Women Walking group joined my monthly walk in central London and what a great pleasure that was. She commented that she felt she had made new friends through sharing the walk together and what we saw, talked about and laughed over.

On the Camino Experiences, I am continually bringing together women from different sides of the Atlantic who form lasting bonds. Because of this campaign, all of us are connecting.

At a recent meeting of my monthly networking group, one of the members stood up and told of a circular she had read, sent round the apartments in her building where one of the women talked about having got involved with a group called One Million Women Walking run by a lady called Heather Waring – my colleague expressed her delight in being able to say 'I know her'. The world is a small place and this campaign is bringing women together through walking.

As I observe the development of the group so far, the women are inspired to walk either more or in some cases to start walking. They are posting in the group regularly, and for some this is daily, which they say helps to keep them on track and focused. Others want to meet walking buddies and in some places that has been happening. A few of the women have shared the wish to undertake a challenge, for example walking the South Downs Way, and want to post in the group so that they are accountable to others and not just themselves and their nearest and dearest. I have had offers of women wanting to become ambassadors, and when I mentioned the Walk

Challenge, a free challenge and group that I was merging with this one, many of the One Million Women wanted to join . There is no shortage of love for this walking activity and its praises are sung daily.

I want to ensure that all this continues and that this community remains vibrant and fulfilling. I also want it to grow further of course. In terms of women, one million is the goal, but it's not just about growing it number wise, it's about what it can achieve and, of course, the impact it can have.

I post questions around a number of things and will be sharing findings. I post what I know is valuable walking information and will be looking at how we can most efficiently manage the group as it continues to grow. I say 'we' because there is more need than ever now to build the team within my business.

In terms of growing numbers, I am looking to raise the group's profile, to get us into the media through articles and interviews in magazines, on blogs and through podcasts. My own podcast is scheduled to launch in 2020, which gives more opportunity to talk about what this initiative means.

I wish to develop an Ambassador Programme as well as a Walk Leader Training with support and ongoing personal growth for leaders as, in that way, One Million Women Walking will provide an infrastructure for the women who are walking already and those who may want to walk. This will start close to home in the UK and Ireland and then expand globally.

In 2020, England's 2800-mile Coastal Path opens. Learning about this has had me thinking of how to mark it, and where WomenWalking:WomenTalking and One Million Women Walking fits. I see a series of events all over the country in perhaps 2021 and/or 2022, bringing women of all ages together through walking. I also see us showcasing all levels of walking, and walking coupled with mindfulness and meditation, as well as with Forest Bathing and a fuller appreciation of nature. I see partnerships and collaboration with organisations and charities concerned with our natural world, sustainability and health and wellbeing.

Moving further forward I am also looking at expanding the bigger view of health and wellbeing including our self-care, because all of these are part of our holistic health, and without health what do we have? That will mean more group and 1-2-1 work often using technology such as zoom and the social media platforms and who knows what else is round the corner to make this work even easier. It's amazing how we can bring together, for a period of an hour or so, a mix of women spread across the globe who share, learn from and support each other in the same way that our geographically close friends do even though they have never met.

As someone who has walked the Camino de Santiago, I was very excited to see that the Pilgrims' Way is considered the UK alternative to that path. However, on starting to walk it, I find myself disappointed and frustrated in equal measure. In Winchester, at the cathedral, which is one of the two main starting points for this major pilgrimage path, there was no sign nor mention of the way at all and in the other, Southwark Cathedral, although we managed to get our Pilgrim passport, there was no indication that it was available. As on the Camino, I want to be able to collect my pilgrim stamps, which along with photos and memories tell the story of my journey. Along the way there are so few churches open, or if they are, you are greeted with blank stares when you inquire about a passport stamp. For this very reason I was jumping with joy, yet a little unbelieving, to discover a stamp in a church in Wrothem, Kent. An absolute joy to see and a reminder that this is not a hard thing to do. There haven't been any others since, apart from the one in Rochester cathedral when we detoured, as many of the Pilgrims did.

Hardly anywhere along the path is there an actual signpost mentioning the Pilgrims' Way. I appreciate that many other shorter walks are along the same trail for differing lengths of distance, but not all who want to walk the Pilgrims' Way are local women who may be familiar with the other named paths. I would argue not having signs doesn't help those who have chosen to walk another of the most famous Pilgrim routes in the world. I feel that this lack puts people off, and with that goes a potential loss of income and jobs

to the area and the loss of the chance to raise the profile of the Pilgrims'
Way. With good signage comes more opportunity to really enjoy the path
and all that there is to be seen, as there is no necessity to burrow your head
in the guide book for fear of missing a turning. I would love to see it elevated
to its rightful place and the infrastructure developed to allow people of all
means to experience it. I feel a call to see what role I can play in doing this.

Who knows what the future might bring and what opportunities will arise?
For me, this mission and campaign is calling me to step up and further into
my role as a leader, a global leader. I am excited to shine the light on this
activity because I fully believe it is revolutionary. I could talk about it for
hours, and my library of books on the subject continues to grow. I am so
grateful for what the wonderful women in this community are bringing to it
and how I am empowering them to step up to and make a difference. Some
have invited all their friends and family, now I am asking them to reach out
further and invite women they come across in their everyday lives. That's one
of the ways we will continue to grow. We truly are more powerful together; so
as you read this, know that you are so important to me.

As I listen to what women are saying, especially about what they want or
need, and I read what they discuss and post as well as what is happening in
the world, ideas flow and possibilities raise their heads. It's important that
there is space for me to experiment and to play, to be spontaneous and to

reach out to others. The feedback this community gives is priceless.

My vision and the legacy just continue to grow, and at times it takes my breath away. It has the potential to be huge, much bigger than I can ever imagine and, of course, that is scary and has me asking questions of myself and my abilities. However, what is the alternative? Just stopping here does not excite and or make me feel good. The adrenaline when I consider the magnitude of what I am creating is what keeps me buzzing.

Burnout and adrenal fatigue were the biggest 'gifts' I could ever have been given. They led me to a bigger self, a greater self with the capacity to bring change to the world. Now there are articles written by GPs (General Practitioners) and MDs (Medical Doctors) talking about how walking affects our health and wellbeing, there are medical papers and research and magazines dedicated to walking and full of its impact. These assist my work so much and I am grateful that the science behind the benefits are starting to be recognised at last and taken seriously.

The time to act is now, and I need you. There is a place for you in working with me to grow this. Together the impact is bigger, stronger and more far-reaching.

Whether it is because you love walking or are intrigued by my story doesn't matter. You are here. What is your story about walking? Is it similar to mine in any way? How does this simple activity impact you?

I would love you to share your stories with me. You can do so through the One Million Women Walking group on Facebook, or you can email me, or we can even have a chat on the phone. You will find my contact details in Appendix 2. Your stories will also inspire, and when you consider a global community like the one I am building here, the more stories from different cultures and different parts of the world, the more value we will add, the more relatable this community will be.

We have a hashtag for this campaign – #onemillionwomenwalking – and I would love you to go on social media as a result of reading this book and use the hashtag #onemillionwomenwalking to tell other women about it. Let them know that this book is here and that they can read it. Share the link to Amazon so that they can get their own copy; tell us all what you liked about it, and how the book or walking has helped you. Let's tell the world about the magic of walking; let's shout its benefits from the rooftops; and let's get more women involved by joining One Million Women Walking – https://www.facebook.com/groups/onemillionwomenwalking/.

If you read the book wherever you are in the world do go on Amazon and post a review. Reviews are of great help to the many women who will come after you who may want to read it but aren't sure. Your words can impact them.

I am not naive enough to think that walking is going to be everyone's chosen form of exercise, and that's fine, but even in a small way it can make a difference. I get some of the greatest joy in my life from seeing women I introduce to walking step into it (no pun intended) and fully embrace it. I see how it changes their lives and impacts it in a range of ways. It doesn't impact everyone in the same way. For some, it de-stresses them, for others it helps with weight loss and reshaping their body, and for others it provides a new interest or hobby and a new community.

Walking has been described as 'medicine for the mind', and I would add, also for the 'soul'.

The first walk that really impacted my life took place on Easter Monday when I was about 15 years old. We, as a family, walked at the Giant's Causeway in Northern Ireland. It was a beautiful day and I vividly remember the colours of the sea, sky and the cliffs. We followed a narrow path that took us along the coast, not far from the water's edge and then, after a few miles, climbed a flight of wooden steps and returned along the top of the cliff by another path. Little did I know on that day just how important walking would become in my life.

I consider myself extremely blessed to be doing what I do and making the difference I make.

Come walk with me, come work with me as, together, we impact those One Million Women.

"The only way to understand a land is to walk it. The only way to drink in its real meaning is to keep it firmly beneath one's feet ... Only the walker can form the wider view"

— Sinclair McKay, Ramble on: The Story of Our Love for Walking Britain

APPENDICES

How to get started

Bringing walking into your life doesn't mean you have to want to hike, trek, tramp or hill-walk along long-distance paths. It's not about rushing around; it's not necessarily about walking many miles, or about how fast you can do it at this stage. It's about what feels good to you and enjoying it.

It can be that regular walk in the local park with your dog, getting together with a friend, or using walking as your way of exploring a new place, be that a beach or a wander through the streets of a city or town. It can be whatever you want, and as much or as little as you choose.

- If you are recovering from burnout, adrenal fatigue, or another illness or injury, or just starting out, then start slowly and build. For some, this might mean just getting out into the garden first or taking a short walk from your front door.

  Ask yourself, how did that feel? This will be your indicator as you build.

- Do the same walk for a day or two and then start to increase your time out walking, and also the distance, but keep it gradual. Keep asking yourself, how did that feel? How do I feel?

- If all this would be made easier by having someone to be accountable to, then go walking with a friend as it's much harder to pull out of the plan when it affects someone else. Or you could be accountable through a friend or loved one by telling them when you plan to walk and then getting them to make sure you do it. You can also use a group like One Million Women Walking for that too –https://www.facebook.com/groups/onemillionwomenwalking/

- Continue to expand your walking. This might be through more days or more times a day or through distance. Again, you get to choose.

- Plan to gather together a few different routes that you can use easily and make them your 'go to' places.

- 'Be' more in the moment as you walk by paying attention to all that is around you. Use your senses to increase your connection to your surroundings and to yourself.

- If it's a horrible cold or wet day, or even a really hot day, and you don't want to be outside, walk round your house or go to a shopping mall. You will be amazed at how many steps you walk. Or go to the gym and use the treadmill. No real substitute for walking in nature but it is better than nothing. Be creative.

How to get involved with me

- Join the Facebook group and help us make that impact –
  https://www.facebook.com/groups/onemillionwomenwalking/

- Use the hashtag #onemillionwomenwalking on social media whenever
  you can.

- Visit my website - **http://1millionwomenwalking.com/** and find out
  everything that I do.

  This site will continue to evolve and to be sure you get all the news and
  opportunities do **join my Inner Circle**

- Download '7 Days of Mindful Walking' -
  http://1millionwomenwalking.com/seven-days-mindful-walking/
  and 'be' in the moment.

- Get yourself a copy of the Walk Your Way Toolkit and create walking
  adventures all year round –
  http://1millionwomenwalking.com/walking-tookit/

Printed in Great Britain
by Amazon